Tuning In

Mindfulness in Teaching and Learning

A collection of essays
for teachers by teachers

Irene McHenry and Richard Brady, Editors

Friends Council on Education

1507 Cherry Street, Philadelphia, PA 19102 • www.friendscouncil.org

Tuning In: Mindfulness in Teaching and Learning
ISBN: 978-0-9824030-0-6

© 2009 by the Friends Council on Education
Irene McHenry and Richard Brady, Editors

*Photographs on the cover and throughout this publication are
from student mandala projects created in Eric Mayer's world religions class
at Westtown School, Pennsylvania.*

Table of Contents

Acknowledgments. 1

Introduction 3

Part I – Teaching Mindfulness 5

Schooled in the Moment
Richard Brady 7

Developing Integrity and Balance
Kimberly Post Rowe. 13

How to Teach Mindfulness Meditation to Children and Beginners
Sumi Loundon Kim 17

Beanie Baby Meditation
Mary Scattergood 33

Muscles, Pebbles, and Good Will
Irene McHenry 37

Learning Silence and Reflection Through the Body: Yoga Class
Barry Blumenfeld 47

Exploring Mindfulness with Elementary School Students
Judy Belasco 51

Part II — Quaker Practices that Center in Mindfulness 57

Meeting for Worship: Developing Reflective Practice
in Friends Schools
Irene McHenry 59

Love, Admiration, and Respect: Meeting for Worship in the Classroom
Christie Duncan-Tessmer 65

How Shall I Use My Time in Meeting for Worship?
Chip Poston. 73

Opening a World of Silence
Mary B. Minor Sidwell 79

The Magic Eye: Tuning In During Meeting for Worship
Richard Brady 81

Worship Sharing: Centering and Reflective Inquiry in Friends Schools
Irene McHenry 83

Mindful Discernment: The Clearness Process
Janet Chance 87

Mindfulness in a School Community
Marcy Baker Seitel 91

Part III — Cultivating Mindful Learning 99

Empty Rooms, Magic Oysters, and Talking Pencils
Rebecca Martin-Scull 101

Nurturing the Inner Garden
Denise Aldridge 107

Writing Is an Act of Love: Mindfulness and Micro-fiction
Hope Blosser 111

"Why Are We Doing This?" Nurturing Academic Mindfulness
Through Self-Grading
Douglas Tsoi 119

Making Sand Mandalas: An Exercise in Impermanence and Letting Go
Eric Mayer 127

Turning Toward the Other: Lectio Divina
Richard Brady 133

A Spinning Top — One Whole Mindful Experience
Daniel Rouse 137

About the Authors 139

References 143

Acknowledgments

Irene McHenry, Executive Director, Friends Council on Education

This book celebrates all teachers who are creatively integrating mindfulness practice into their daily endeavors in school communities around the world. The wide-ranging explorations of mindfulness experience highlighted in this collection arise from the authors' deep wells of creativity, careful response to students' needs, and disciplined practice in the art and science of mindfulness.

I am indebted to Shinzen Young, who helped me see that mindfulness practice develops a powerful foundation for all teaching and learning – the core skills of concentration, observation, relaxation and empathy. I extend profound gratitude to co-editor Richard Brady for his inspired work and for his model of living a life grounded in mindful attention and loving kindness. Richard and I cherish Thich Nhat Hanh's compassionate teachings, engaged social activism and abundant creativity in making mindfulness accessible across many religions and cultures; and, we greatly appreciate Jon Kabat-Zinn's leading work in mindfulness-based stress reduction and research that brings mindfulness into the mainstream of medicine, psychology and education. This book was made possible by the steadfast commitment, skill, and guidance of the Friends Council's Associate Director Sarah Sweeney-Denham, the passion and talent of production editor Nancy Adess, and the dedicated work of volunteer extraordinaire Mary Hanisch.

Thank you to all teachers, learners, and researchers working to expand the application and benefits of mindfulness in education, and to you, the readers of this book. Wherever you begin, I hope that *Tuning In* encourages investigation combined with disciplined practice, fresh insights leading to possibilities, and that it motivates your taking time and space in every day to stop, breathe, and expand our interconnected capacity for wholeness.

Introduction

The seed for this book was planted eight years ago when we began our work together creating Mindfulness for Educators workshops with the goal of sharing mindfulness practices with teachers, administrators, school counselors, and others working with children, adolescents and adults in their school communities. Richard was teaching mindfulness to ninth graders at Sidwell Friends School as a means of stress reduction. Irene was using mindfulness practices with young children, teens and adults in her psychotherapy practice and teaching seventh graders at the William Penn Charter School how to use meditation techniques for centering and quiet focusing during weekly Meeting for Worship.

The essays in this collection vividly demonstrate that contemplative methods can be used with any curriculum content to support capacity development for self-understanding, empathy, emotional intelligence and social skills. These experientially-based vignettes show children, teenagers and teachers using pebbles, mandalas, literature, beanie babies, yoga, journals, homework, artwork to strengthen the core skills underlying all learning: concentration, observation, relaxation, and open, receptive awareness with a positive, curious attitude. This pedagogy teaches children a new way to think, to learn, and to know, leading to the development of critical thinking and the valuing of multiple perspectives, the capacity to solve problems and the motivation to do so as members of their local and the world community. "The basic ingredients of well-being and compassionate social living are, in fact, teachable. Reflection is the common pathway by which our brains support such abilities" (Siegel, 2007).

The Friends Council on Education is honored to contribute this publication to the growing field of literature on the value and essential utility of mindfulness skills and practice in educational settings to benefit teaching and learning at all levels. The recent explosion of mindfulness resources in our culture comes from the intersection of ancient mindfulness practices from the East, contemplative practices from the early Greeks, and current research on brain neuroplasticity in the West. This synergy and momentum for bringing mindfulness into education is informed by research on mindful awareness, creativity, and problem solving with teachers and students in public and private schools. Research demonstrates that optimal learning occurs when the

mind is relaxed and alert, fully open to itself and the external world
(Siegel, 2007). Mindfulness methods and related practices in education
are frequently described with two umbrella terms: contemplative
education and mindfulness. Contemplative education refers to
education that employs "a third way of knowing that complements
the rational and the sensory" (Hart, 2004). Contemplative methods
encourage reflective inquiry, curiosity, and discovery; contemplative
learning requires patience. Contemplative methods complement left-
brain linear, logical thinking by opening the creative right-brain channels
for intuitive insight, fresh observations, creative understanding, and
deep knowing. A simple operational definition of mindfulness comes
from the mindfulness-based stress reduction work of Kabat-Zinn (2005).
Mindfulness is the awareness that comes from developing the skillset of
paying attention, on purpose and without judgment, to the experience in
each immediate moment as it unfolds.

The practical illustrations in this collection of essays are primarily from
teachers' work with children and teens in grades K-12. Richard and I are
grateful for the many opportunities to explore new classroom practices
over the years with teachers and students in public and private schools,
as well as higher education. We thank not only the contributors to this
book, but also the many educators and counselors that inspired each
other during periods of meditation practice in our workshops and
through sharing their energy and ideas for cultivating mindfulness in
the classroom and in school communities.

Editors:

Irene McHenry, Ph.D., Executive Director,
Friends Council on Education

Richard Brady, M.S., Mindfulness Consultant and Teacher

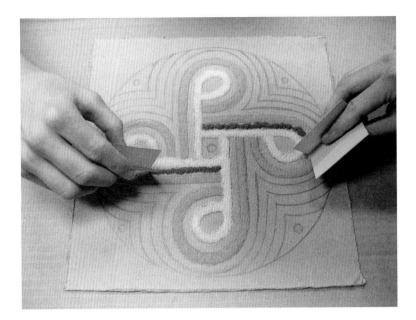

PART I
Teaching Mindfulness

Mindfulness practices can be taught to students of all ages to help them settle and center, sharpen awareness, and reduce stress. In this section teachers describe using practices that ground their students in awareness of the present moment by focusing on sensory input from the body and from emotions.

Kimberly Post Rowe provides an introduction to the benefits of mindfulness for both teachers and students, and introduces walking meditation as a mindfulness practice. Sumi Kim asks her seventh- and eighth-grade students to begin their experience of centering by simply listening to sounds in their environment. She then invites them to investigate taste, eating in a meditative manner. Finally, she uses body relaxation as preparation for focusing on breath, teaching awareness of the breath as a foundation for body awareness. Similarly, Irene McHenry and Richard Brady use breath as the basis for body relaxation practices. Body-centered mindfulness can also be developed through chanting and yoga, as described by Barry Blumenfeld. Mary Scattergood engages second-graders in awareness of the breath by using their special objects—Beanie Babies. Judy Belasco uses a singing bowl to focus her students' attention.

The practice of metta, or good will, which focuses students' attention on love, is another tool, described in this section by McHenry, Kim, and Blumenthal. Thoughts, as well as emotions, bodily sensations, and sensory input, are all components of the "Stage of Awareness" experiment Brady uses to introduce mindfulness to his students.

Many of these techniques appear again in the context of cultivating mindful learning and relationships in Part III.

Schooled in the Moment: Introducing Mindfulness to High School Students and Teachers

Richard Brady

I grew up on Chicago's north shore, the area, I later learned, that had the highest teenage suicide rate in the country at the time. My own high school years were uneventful, but my younger brother's were very troubled. I suspect his unhappiness was a major reason for my choosing to devote my life to working with teenagers. After teaching high school mathematics for 30 years, I realized that there was something more I needed to be doing with my life. I took a year off from teaching to explore the possibilities, but within a few weeks I had my answer. A friend called to tell me about the tensions students and teachers were experiencing in schools in her area. "Someone should teach them meditation," I heard myself reply. Immediately, it dawned on me: I was that someone. I soon found support for my decision in Jon Kabat-Zinn's *Full Catastrophe Living*.

During the last three years, returning to school, I have been given a number of opportunities to introduce mindfulness practice to students and teachers in my Quaker high school as well as to student and faculty groups in other private and public high schools. I usually advertise my presentations under the banner of "stress reduction," since this is a fairly widespread issue for both high school students and faculty. Several major premises underlie these presentations: high school students and teachers are seldom aware of how their minds work; when given the opportunity to see how their minds work, they enjoy doing so; the experience will, in many cases, reveal sources of stress that meditation can alleviate.

The "Stage" of Awareness

When I present mindfulness workshops to students and high school teachers, I begin by suggesting that our minds play a significant role in our well-being. When I talk about mind, I say, I am talking about awareness. I then lead an experience to give people an understanding of what I mean. I suggest that it helps to think of one's awareness as a

7

theater stage. On that stage a succession of things make an appearance: thoughts, feelings, perceptions, physical sensations. I tell the group that we will conduct a short experiment so that we can watch what is playing on our personal stages. I ask them to get comfortable in their seats and then to close their eyes and tune in to whatever may be on their stages of awareness. I ask them simply to try to watch whatever thoughts, feelings, perceptions, and sensations arise during the next few minutes, observing them, but not getting carried away by them.

After five minutes I ask them to slowly open their eyes. Then I ask them to respond to a series of questions by raising their hands: How many were aware of physical sensations—sounds, smells, tastes, contact with the seat, their heartbeat, their breathing, their feet, and so on? How many were aware of their emotions or thoughts? How many saw a thought arise? A thought end? Regarding feelings, I ask how many people experienced negative, neutral, or positive feelings? Of the negative feelings, how many had to do with things that have already happened, things they're feeling upset or guilty about? Usually quite a few relate to this question. I then ask how many negative thoughts and feelings had to do with the future, things they are anxious about? This also gets a substantial response. Finally, I ask how many negative thoughts and feelings had to do with the present?

Ultimately, I point out that what our minds do during this particular five-minute interval of our waking life is repeated about 70,000 times each year. If we multiply the number of negative thoughts and feelings we observed by 70,000, we might understand why the mind plays such a significant role in creating stress. However, if we are able to become more aware of the negative thoughts and feelings that enter our minds and develop ways to replace them with positive ones, we will be able to live happier, less stressful lives—in school and beyond. Meditation, I explain, is one way to help our minds respond to negative thinking in a healthy way.

My Experience of Learning to Meditate

When I started reading *The Miracle of Mindfulness* by Vietnamese Buddhist monk Thich Nhat Hanh 15 years ago, I found the teaching so compelling that I began each math class with a short reading from the book. The students greatly appreciated the instructions for living more focused, peaceful lives they found in the readings. When we finished that book, I went on to read from another of his books, *The Sun My Heart*. The mindful way of living portrayed by Thich Nhat Hanh in these books sounded great. However, it felt so different from my own that it seemed to me that I could not get there from where I was.

As fate would have it, near the end of that school year, when the seniors returned from three weeks off-campus working on senior projects, I heard a presentation by one of the seniors—a boy named Chris—about his project at the Zen Center of Washington, D.C. Chris began by telling us that a classmate and he had been reading Eastern religion and philosophy since seventh grade. Recently, he had discovered the local Zen center and "decided to put my body where my mind was." I felt Chris talking directly to me.

He spoke of his experience with tremendous enthusiasm. He showed pictures and recounted some dramatic experiences during the three-day intensive meditation retreat he attended as part of his project. At the conclusion of his talk, another student asked Chris whether his life was different in any way besides doing a lot of sitting on cushions now. Chris responded by saying that meditation had many effects on him. "However," he added, "most are so subtle I can't put them into words." After a pause, he went on, "I can tell you that I am less angry." Chris's presentation, especially this last statement, was very moving to me. I thanked him and made a promise to him and to myself that I would try to meditate.

During the following six years I met Thich Nhat Hanh, began a daily meditation practice, helped establish the Washington Mindfulness Community, which supported this practice, and attended two retreats in Plum Village, Thich Nhat Hanh's monastic community in southwestern France. On returning from my second retreat to Plum Village, I gave an assembly at my high school about my experiences, which included stories about Plum Village life and a slide show. At the close of the assembly I led a brief meditation focused on the breath.

A few days after the Plum Village assembly, as our high school sat in its weekly Quaker Meeting, a senior named Audrey rose and spoke out. She told the students how, late the previous night, closing her eyes and focusing on her breath had dispelled her feelings of stress. She concluded, "The action is so little, but the reward is tremendous."

A Guided Meditation

When I give presentations now, I include Chris', Audrey's, and my stories because they provide a good opportunity for me to invite the participants to move, as I did, from learning about meditation to practicing it. I then lead the group in a 10-minute guided meditation, using Thich Nhat Hanh's mindfulness verse (or gatha):

In/Out
Deep/Slow
Calm/Ease
Smile/Release
Present Moment/Wonderful Moment

To prepare the group for the meditation, I ask them to sit erect, shoulders relaxed, both feet on the floor. Then I ask them to focus on their breath and to coordinate their in and out breaths with the phrases of the meditation verse. I use a bell to begin and end the meditation and to signal each transition. At the conclusion of the meditation, I ask the participants to turn to a neighbor and share their experience. Sometimes this involves waking up a fellow student or teacher.

This short introduction seems to convey the importance of awareness of the mind. I've encountered a variety of reactions. In one faculty workshop a teacher told me, "I could not even begin to focus on my breath and the words you gave me because I'm so riled up about an encounter I just had with a student." This is one of many possible meditations, I replied. The breath can also assist us in being with strong emotions, helping us hold them in our awareness without getting lost in them. However, our meditation practice needs to be strong in order to use it that way. If we are able to embrace our emotions with our breath, we may learn some valuable things about ourselves and relate to our emotions in a less stressful way in the process.

Concentration and Dealing with Difficult Emotions

The members of the Physical Education Department at my school were not able to come to my meditation assembly, so they invited me to run a special workshop for them. I started in a similar fashion, inviting them to observe their minds. Then, since the group was interested in developing concentration in their sports teams and it was lunchtime, I invited them to do eating meditation with raisins. Later the boys' varsity basketball coach asked if there might be something I could do with his team members to improve their foul shooting. A week later, I was with the team as they stood in a row facing a basket, each with a basketball in hand. I explained that we would do a meditation that could help them focus on the shot they were about to make and not be distracted by the noise of the fans. I then asked the players to assume comfortable positions with eyes closed and, when I blew the coach's whistle, to begin watching whatever was passing through their awareness and continue doing this until I blew the whistle a second time, after five minutes. I didn't have the opportunity to get the players' reactions, but I heard later that the team's foul shooting improved.

Several years ago a religion teacher at another Quaker school invited me to share mindfulness practice with a twelfth-grade class studying the Holocaust. The class had been focusing on events leading up to the Holocaust and would soon be reading disturbing, graphic accounts of the Holocaust itself. To help prepare the students to be open to the suffering they would be encountering, I told them that mindfulness practice could provide a way to be with suffering without being overwhelmed by it. I described the process of holding emotions in one's awareness like a mother cradling a crying infant, holding the emotions with great tenderness. Class members then chose personal experiences of "suffering" out of their own lives, something they could relate to, such as an argument with a friend or a low test grade. After leading a guided meditation that helped them focus awareness on their breath, I asked them to bring their suffering into their awareness and hold it gently for five minutes. Afterward, some students responded to my invitation to share their experiences with the class.

Deepening the Observation

Over the last few years how I teach mindfulness to students and teachers has changed as my own understanding and practice of mindfulness have been affected by it. I first approached students with the notion that negative thoughts and feelings not only lead to stress, but were intrinsically bad. Watching negativity was part of my sales pitch for the guided meditation to follow, which had the potential for changing the mind's channel away from negative thoughts and emotions. Now I find sitting back and just watching whatever is on stage important in and of itself—whether negative or positive. I now explain to students that to the extent that they are able to watch their stage without engaging, they will have less need to tune in to a different show. They can begin to see both negative and positive scenes as transitory products of mind and simply be with them, understanding that their primary significance lies in what you make of them. So I no longer present the guided relaxation meditation as the only means of responding to negative mind states.

My foremost goal in teaching—whether meditation or mathematics—is the same: to offer my students opportunities to be mindful of their minds, of their breath, of mathematics and math problems, of other students, and of their own ways of learning. As I create opportunities for mindfulness, students discover the meaning and value of their own experiences for themselves.

This essay is adapted from an article that appeared in Independent School Magazine, *Fall 2004.*

Developing Integrity and Balance

Kimberly Post Rowe

As holistic educator Jack Miller noted more than a decade ago, "We live in what has been called the age of alienation.… We tend to live in a world that is fragmented, and our lives are filled with the experience of separateness." Pulled in many directions at once, we are expected to multitask constantly, leaving little time for personal pursuits or quiet introspection. Multitasking is a chronic side effect of our modern lives. Most of us have been taught that there is nothing wrong with it (we are merely being efficient), and there is nothing wrong with pondering (read: fretting) about the future (we are merely being forward-looking). But in actuality, we might question the benefits of such efficiency and the outcomes of our fretting. In our daily struggle to be globally competitive, absorb ever-larger amounts of information, and be effective parents, spouses, children, employees, and friends, we have become startlingly out of balance. Our outer lives seem to demand all of our attention, while our inner lives are increasingly left behind.

Ralph Waldo Emerson often reflected on the importance of an inner life: "What lies before us and what lies behind us are tiny matters compared to what lies within us," he said. But for most of us, taking the time to cultivate an inner life seems selfish and self-centered. To further complicate matters, the introspection and self-examination required for developing a balanced inner life pose a risk. What if, upon quiet reflection, we find that our true selves don't jibe with all of those external expectations? How can we live with integrity?

The term "integrity" does not only mean being true to our beliefs. Dictionaries define integrity as "being whole or undivided." Indeed, living with integrity is a regular concern voiced by educators. Many feel that the current educational climate is creating a schism, effectively removing the heart and soul from pedagogy as increasing expectations dictate discounting the personal needs and interests of students in favor of developing their global competitiveness. In *The Courage to Teach*, Parker Palmer goes so far as to say that "good teaching comes from the…integrity of the teacher."

Perhaps this is the real reason that we are struggling with a lack of balance in our lives. As teachers, how can we reunite our inner sense of truth and integrity with our outward behavior? How can we rejoin *soul* with *role*? We need to reclaim our integral balance and find what Palmer calls our "hidden wholeness."

We need to shift our perspective. If we *take the time* to tend our inner landscapes, to allow our inner truth to find expression and value in our outer lives, then we are not being selfish—we are increasing our potential to be generous. We will be infinitely more effective and present as parents, spouses, children, employees, and friends. The practice of bringing our inner selves into balance can enable us to function with integrity, as whole human beings, and so bring our external lives into balance as well.

During the 1995 State of the World Forum in San Francisco, Zen Buddhist monk, teacher, and author Thich Nhat Hanh spoke of mindfulness as a powerful tool for strengthening relationships and personal connections, as quoted in an article about the Forum in *Shambhala Sun*:

> Today, communication has expanded greatly throughout the world. Email, fax, voice pager — you can contact New York from Tokyo in half a minute so easily. Yet in families and in neighborhoods, between husbands and wives, between friends and each other, real communication is still difficult....We need to rediscover a way to talk and listen to each other as in a loving family. But what technology can help with this? I feel the need is for practice, for mindful listening. A heart free to listen is a flower that blooms on the tree of practice.

"A heart free to listen." Thich Nhat Hanh teaches that mindfulness encourages us to be thoughtful, present, and capable of deep listening— qualities needed in all healthy relationships. Practicing mindfulness helps to develop intuition, intentionality, self-control, and awareness of personal values. In a nutshell, mindfulness begets integral balance.

In the fifth installation of the Star Wars saga, *The Empire Strikes Back*, Jedi master Yoda tells Luke Skywalker why he is not well-suited to becoming a Jedi: "A Jedi must have the deepest commitment, the most serious mind. This one a long time have I watched. All his life has he looked away...to the future, to the horizon. Never his mind on where he was." At first glance, it seems as if Yoda is implying that Luke is a daydreamer, lazy and driven by childish notions of adventure. But he is actually saying that being present in the moment — being mindful — is of utmost importance.

Whether we aspire to be Jedi masters or merely to live more balanced lives, developing a mindfulness practice may be the most important thing we can do to cultivate a rich inner life and deepen our connections with others. It is done by bringing the mind to focus on what is happening in the present moment. Contemplative prayer, hiking, painting, even cooking can all be tools for developing mindfulness when done with intention.

Walking is an ideal activity to begin to bring mindfulness into one's everyday life. Walking in a mindful, meditative way heightens your attention to the details of sound, touch, smell, and sight of all that's around you. Following are the instructions I use when I introduce walking meditation to students and teachers. While specific to walking, the spirit of these instructions can be applied to any activity—eating, cleaning, even working on or grading homework.

Walking Meditation

Begin by closing your eyes and listening. *(Pause for a few breaths.)* Sounds are layered all around us. As you notice one sound, take a moment to really listen to it before putting it aside to make room for another. *(Pause for a few breaths.)* You may notice that sometimes a word or phrase springs to mind when you identify yet another sound. Other times you may feel a sound in your body, experiencing a jolt of recognition or an emotional reaction to what you are hearing. *(Pause for a few breaths.)* Try to listen without judging—no blame, no praise, just listening.

Take a few deep breaths of air and notice the sounds your body makes. Breathe in through your nose so that you can smell the freshness of the air around you, and exhale out through your mouth so you can listen to the air leave your body. *(Pause for a few breaths.)* As you listen to your body, you may begin to notice the many scents moving through the air around you. *(Pause for a breath.)* Sometimes the air is so redolent, you can almost taste it on your tongue.

Feel the air against your skin. Notice the temperature, the movement. Can you hear the air as it moves? Does it make a sound for your ears or is it more of a vibration dancing on the surface of your skin? *(Pause for a few breaths.)* Feel the ground beneath your feet. Does it feel firm or soft, smooth or uneven?

Keep your attention on your feet and let your eyes open to a soft focus. Do you still sense the surface beneath your feet? *(Pause for a breath.)* Keeping your awareness on the places where your feet make contact with the ground, begin to walk. Go slowly, noticing the exaggerated sensation that heightened awareness brings to your stride—each heel planting to the ground ahead, rolling to toe, and lifting to plant again.

Now, listen to the sounds your feet make as they crunch on the ground. You may be surprised at how loud your steps seem, and how the sound of your steps adds another layer of sound to the air around you. *(Pause.)* Continue to walk at this slower pace, paying attention to the many sounds, taking the time to really listen to each one before putting it aside to make room for another. *(Pause.)* Notice how each sound seems to take on a life of its own as you bring your attention to it.

As you walk, begin to observe the sights around you. Use your eyes to explore your walking. Notice the ground beneath you, the colors, the shifting shadows. *(Pause.)* Allow your eyes to wander over the many surfaces, noticing the textures, the changing landscape, as you slowly continue to place one foot in front of the other. *(Pause.)* When you use your eyes in this way, noticing the many variations of color, the play of light and shadow, your heightened awareness allows you to appreciate the beauty of each detail, each moment, each breath.

We will continue to walk in silence—no spoken words now. Notice when you are recognizing a sound, or when you deeply breathe a scent as it wafts by. *(Pause.)* Notice when you are using your eyes to appreciate your walking experience, and when you feel your body shift as it moves through the air and makes contact with the surface beneath you. *(Pause.)* There is plenty of time—every detail, every experience is of equal importance.

How to Teach Mindfulness Meditation to Children and Beginners

Sumi Loundon Kim

How can you, as a teacher, introduce young people the basics of mindfulness meditation? What can you say, what should you have the children do?

The following program can be done in a period as short as one and one-half hours or as long as three hours. I have used the same program with children as young as six, as well as with teens, college students, parents, and teachers, increasing the duration of each exercise, and thus the length of the program overall, with the age of the group. The version outlined here is designed for seventh- and eighth-graders in a public school setting. Thus, the language here is simple and there are no references to the Buddhist tradition from which mindfulness meditation is drawn.

Program Overview

Mindfulness of Hearing: "How Many Sounds" Contest
Mindfulness of Tasting: Raisin Meditation
Mindfulness of Movement I: Palms Together
Mindfulness of Movement II: Walking Meditation

Stretch and/or Break

Mindfulness of Body: Full-Body Relaxation and Stress Release
Mindfulness of Breath
Opening the Heart: Loving kindness Meditation

Method: Children find it challenging to take the breath as the initial object of meditation because the sensations of the breath are subtle. To help children learn how to be mindful of the many qualities of an experience, therefore, it is better to begin with more easily perceived sensations. For example, chewing a raisin slowly engages taste, texture, tongue movement, and the sound of chewing. After cultivating basic skills in observing sensations at finer and finer levels, you can then move to the breath. It is especially effective to do a full-body relaxation first, followed immediately by seated breathing meditation. With the body completely calm and relaxed, the myriad sensations of the breath become readily apparent.

Introduction

Let me ask you: What is meditation all about? It's very popular these days: we hear about the Zen of basketball, movie stars say they do meditation, magazines have articles about stress reduction. But what, really, is meditation?

I like to think of it this way: we clean our rooms, we take showers to clean dirt off our bodies, we brush our teeth—but when do we clean our minds from the clutter of thoughts? When do we intentionally let go of all the stress, anxiety, busy thoughts, memories, and emotions that build up over a day and over weeks? Meditation is like cleaning out the mind. It's like taking a rest in a clear, quiet, calm space.

In order to do meditation, we need to calm our minds down. Our mind is like a puppy. How many of you have had a puppy? As you know, trying to get a puppy to stay in one spot is quite a challenge. You've got the puppy sitting there, panting, wagging its tail, and suddenly it sees a butterfly and it goes dashing off. You bring the puppy back and it sits again. But in half a second it sees a bone over in the grass and goes running off again. You bring it back. The mind is like a puppy because sights, sounds, and even thoughts are constantly distracting it. So we're going to train the puppy mind to calmly stay in one place.

Before we start, I'd like to ask two things from you. First, I expect your 100 percent participation in each activity we do. Second, I want you to respect the time and space of the people around you by refraining from whispering to them, poking them, passing notes, and so on. I thank you for both these things.

Mindfulness of Hearing: "How Many Sounds" Contest

Each student will need a piece of paper, folded in half, and a pen or pencil, plus something hard to write on if the floor is carpeted.

The first exercise is a contest. I'd like to see who can hear the most sounds in one minute. We're going to close our eyes and listen as carefully as possible. When I call "time," open your eyes and then write down each sound you heard.

I. Okay, everyone, close your eyes. *[Minute passes.]* Open your eyes. Without talking, write down everything you heard. After you're done, number the sounds down the side. Who got more than five sounds? More than ten? *[Have the person with the largest list read his or hers aloud. Ask others if they noticed anything else.]*

II. Let's do it again. Close your eyes, and for one minute, listen for as many sounds as you can. *[Minute passes.]* Open your eyes. Again, write down everything you heard and number them. How many of you have a second list that's longer than the first one? *[Nearly everyone will.]* Would someone like to read his or her list?

III. Lesson: Wonderful. Isn't it amazing that almost every person heard more sounds the second time around? Is that because there were more sounds to be heard in the second minute as opposed to the first? No. You heard more sounds the second minute because your ability to listen improved.

You see, mindfulness is like a muscle: the more you exercise it, the stronger it gets. You managed to improve your ability to perceive sounds in just *one* minute. Isn't that amazing? And, you know, this attention muscle is the same muscle that does the heavy lifting of figuring out math problems, writing a paper, and playing baseball. If you practice meditation regularly, you'll find your attention is stronger when you study, when you do sports, when you practice playing an instrument or doing art, and so on.

Mindfulness of Tasting: Raisin Meditation

Each student needs two raisins. Remind students not to eat the raisins until you say so.

I. We've just brought our attention to our sense of hearing, and now we're going to bring it to our sense of taste. In this exercise, we're going to chew one of the raisins as slowly as possible, and when I say slowly, I mean veeeery slowly, like for at least three minutes. When you chew it, I'd like you to notice all the qualities of eating the raisin, from its texture, to its taste, to how your tongue, teeth and other parts of your mouth experience eating it. Okay, put one raisin in your mouth and close your eyes. Go ahead and start observing as you chew. *[Generally, students will take about four minutes with the raisin. Stop the exercise when it seems like a majority of the students have swallowed.]* Okay, go ahead and swallow the raisin if you haven't already, noticing what it's like to swallow, and then open your eyes. So, what kinds of experiences did you have with the raisin? *[Depending on group size, you can go around in a circle, or you can have kids volunteer.]* By the way, guess how long you chewed that raisin for? One minute? Two? No! You chewed it for four minutes! *[The kids will be amazed.]* Isn't it amazing how our perception of time changes when we're really paying attention? Even though we're slowing down, it feels like time passes more quickly.

II. Let's do it again. This time, I want you to think of your mind as a microscope, and I want you to see how strongly your microscope can magnify your experience of eating the raisin. While you're chewing this raisin, try to get down to the smallest particle of sensation. I want you to be like a scientist, looking for the tiniest atom of raisin-chewing experience. Now, take the second raisin in your fingers, close your eyes, but *don't eat the raisin yet*. Instead, bring your awareness to your mouth: can you feel your mouth preparing itself for the sweetness? I just felt my mouth water. Now bring the raisin to your mouth. *[chewing time]* Okay, go ahead and swallow the raisin if you haven't already, noticing what it's like to swallow, and then open your eyes. This time I'd like to hear about the tiniest and perhaps most surprising experience you had with eating the raisin.

III. **Lesson:** Isn't it amazing that something as simple as chewing one single raisin with full attentiveness can open up an entire world of sensation? Imagine eating an entire meal this way! Okay, what can we learn from this? I'd like you to remember the last time you had, say, a scoop of your favorite ice cream. Someone tell me what your favorite kind of ice cream is: (chocolate, vanilla, etc.). Great. So there you are with a scoop of your favorite ice cream, and the first bite— isn't the first bite just so wonderful? It just explodes in your mouth, all that sweetness and cold and melting. But, then, think about the last bite of ice cream. Are you even aware of the ice cream by then? Somehow, as you dug through the ice cream, you got distracted. Maybe you were watching TV or you were talking to someone. The initial burst of sensation of the first spoonful of ice cream has diminished to the point where we're not even aware of the ice cream any more. But, if you bring mindfulness to your experience, you can enjoy the last bite of ice cream as much as the first, and all the bites in between. This way, you can keep your life simple: you don't need an entire banana split to get the same wonderful taste from the ice cream if you are totally mindful of the pleasure that one scoop can bring. In fact, I bet you will feel more satisfied, more fulfilled from eating one scoop mindfully than from eating a whole banana split mindlessly. What this means is that mindfulness can help us regulate our consumption, not just with food but also with video games, movies, or anything that we consume for pleasure.

Note: A student may volunteer that he or she does not like raisins, which presents a wonderful opportunity to make a valuable point. That is, that we can be mindful of unpleasant experiences as much as we are of pleasant experiences. *All* experience is available for mindfulness practice. Moreover, when we observe our experience carefully, we may be able to distinguish between the actual experience of tasting the raisin versus the mental activity of disliking or judging the raisin. This kind of distinction is useful when we experience pain, for example: there's the physical sensation of pain and then there is our fear, anxiety, and other thoughts and emotions in reaction to the pain.

Mindfulness of Movement I: Palms Together

Have students pair off and sit facing each other. Each student will need a sheet of paper and pen.

Now that we brought our attention to hearing and tasting, we'll look at the experience of moving our bodies. In this activity, we're going to bring our mindfulness to movement. One person is going to do a simple movement and verbally report on all the sensations of that movement to the other person. The other person is going to be the secretary, writing down what you say. The movement we're going to do is to bring our hands from resting on the knees up to a palms-together position in front of our chests. [*Teacher should demonstrate and verbalize: I feel the warmth of my palms on my knees (the secretary can write down "warmth of palms on knees"). Now I feel my biceps contracting. I feel the cool air under my palms as I lift them in the air. I feel my fingers coming together. . . .] Move very slowly so that you can feel as many sensations as possible.

[*Activity usually takes 10 minutes.*] Who would like to read the movement journal of their partner? [*Someone reads.*] Would anyone else like to share? Okay, let's switch roles. The other person is the secretary and the one who was the secretary can be the person doing the movement. [*Repeat sharing. Reports will usually be more detailed the second time around.*]

Mindfulness of Movement II: Walking Meditation

If time is short, forego this activity. If the space is small, do the walking meditation in a circle with you in the lead and setting the pace. However, if there's enough space, have students walk in their own six- to ten-foot lane. With shoes off, students can feel their feet and the floor more sensitively. If you have lots of time, then it's ideal to start with a moderate walking pace in which students notice gross movements, and then slow the pace down so they can notice finer movements and sensations. In the last few minutes, students can move extremely slowly, noticing micro-movements and sensations. This activity works best if the teacher demonstrates slow walking meditation, verbalizing the experiences. It's also good to remind students that they are not trying to get anywhere.

Teacher can guide by asking questions throughout: What part of the foot leaves the floor last? What part of the foot comes to the floor first? Can you feel your toes spreading as you put more weight on the foot? Now it's time to end: everyone come to a standing position, and just feel yourself standing.

Stretching Out

If you've spent a lot of time on the first set of exercises, it is a good idea to have students take a five- or ten-minute break and then regroup by doing some stretching out together. If you don't have time for a break, then go right to stretching out.

You've done very well, and I especially appreciate your full participation in everything we've done so far. We have really built up our attention muscle! But now, let's take a moment to stretch out and get some energy back in our bodies.

- Reach up to the sky, up on our tippy tippy toes, like a tree, reaching higher, higher, so tall, everything tall reach, reach, reach—and relax.

- Let's stretch out our legs. Curl over slowly until your hands get near the floor. It's okay to bend your knees. Just hanging out here for a moment. Good. And slowly roll up, allowing one vertebra to stack on the next until you come back to standing.

- Let's open up our chest area. Bring your hands behind you and grasp them together. Lift your hands up to the ceiling, opening the chest, don't be shy.

- Let's roll our head around, slowly, loosening the neck.
- Finally, let's shake out our hands. Loose-y goose-y. Let that shake travel up to your arms, then to your shoulders. Let's go to the feet, shake the feet, now let it travel up into your legs, and then into your hips, up to your chest, shoulders, down through the arms and finally the head. Okay, stop. Take a few deep breaths, feeling the body as it rests. Let's sit down again.

Mindfulness of Body: Full Relaxation and De-Stressing

Now we're ready for our next exercise. So far we have brought our attention to sound, then to taste, and then to the motion of our hands coming together and to walking. Now we're going to bring our attention into our bodies and intentionally relax each part of the body, releasing any built-up stress and tension.

Our minds are not separate from our bodies: when our mind is tense and full of busy thoughts, our body becomes tense and stressed out. Likewise, when we relax the body, that sends a message to the mind to relax, to slow down. As your body relaxes, you'll find that your mind softens and relaxes, too. We're going to lie down on the floor, but before we do that, I want you to watch me for a moment. This is how I want you to position your body, on your back, feet slightly apart and falling to the sides, arms away from the body, palms up, head centered. If this is hard on your lower back, you can bend your knees.

I'm going to take you through the full relaxation, and when I'm done, we're going to slowly move into the final exercise, the breathing meditation. This is how I want you to do it. You will very slowly roll over to one side, paying attention to how your body feels. Then make a pillow with your hands and rest there for a moment. Then, I will instruct you to very slowly push up into a sitting position. Keep your eyes to yourself and keep your attention on how your body feels as it moves. When you come to a comfortable sitting position, close your eyes and I'll begin leading you through a breathing meditation. It's very important that you keep your motion to a minimum so that the body and mind can stay in this quiet, rested space for as long as possible.

So, everyone find a spot on the floor and lie down on your back. No need to engage with your friends at this point, no need to talk to anyone. Please respect each other by not touching or poking. Lie down with your legs and arms flat on the floor. The palms of your hands are facing upward toward the ceiling. Let the feet fall away to the sides, allowing your entire body to just fall into the floor. Close your eyes and mouth and bring your attention into your body. Feel the contact of your body with the floor, the hardness, the coldness, the warmth, whatever you feel. *[Depending on how much time you have, you can do large chunks of the body or small parts; for example, the entire foot versus the toes, foot, and ankle.]*

Bring your attention to your feet and consciously relax all the muscles. Completely letting go of any strain, feeling the muscles become soft and relaxed. Now feel the muscles in your calves, letting go of any tightness, allowing the muscles to become soft and relaxed. *[Your voice should soften, become rhythmic in speech]*

[There are actually a variety of relaxation methods. One is autosuggestion: "My feet are relaxing, my feet are relaxing, my feet are relaxed." If you are familiar with a technique from yoga classes, use that. Anything will work! Move to knees, thighs, bottom, pelvis, back, abdomen, chest, down one arm to the hand and then down the other, the shoulders, neck, back of the head, area around the mouth, cheeks, area around the eyes, top of the head, the whole head. Minimum 15 minutes of full relaxation.]

Now let your awareness spread throughout your entire body, allowing every part to completely relax, becoming heavy, soft, falling into the floor. *[Be silent for a few more minutes, letting the children be in their bodies. Many will fall asleep, which is fine.]*

Now, let's re-awaken our bodies by gently moving the fingers. No need to talk or interact with your friends, just stay inside yourself. Gently wiggle the toes. Move your head slowly from side to side. Now slowly roll over onto your left side. Take a rest there, making a pillow with your hands under your head, just feeling how calm and relaxed you feel. Now slowly push yourself up into a sitting position. Please respect others by not interacting with them, just stay inside yourself. *[For those who've fallen asleep, have an assistant teacher gently wake them up.]*

And now come into a sitting position, close your eyes, and feel your whole body, how relaxed it is. *[Teacher should keep voice soft, sitting still in similar position to model for children. Move right into next activity, following.]*

Mindfulness of Breath

Feel your body, feel your bottom touching the floor, your ankles touching the floor and your calf. Feel your hands resting on your knees. Let your awareness be in your entire body, just moving from sensation to sensation. *[Pause for a minute or two.]*

And now bring your awareness into your tummy area, feeling it move as you breathe. Rise and fall. Expanding and contracting. In and out. *[Give students some time to experience this, maybe a minute.]*

Moving your awareness into your chest, feeling it rise and fall, expand and contract, as you breathe. No need to control the breath. Just let it come and go as it will. Sometimes the breath will be long, sometimes short, sometimes deep, sometimes shallow. Just let it be and watch. *[Pause.]*

Moving your awareness to the back of the throat, feeling the air pass there, very soft and gentle, warm and cool, dry and moist. *[Pause.]*

Moving your awareness to the back of the nose area, feeling the air passing in and out, warm and cool, dry and moist, in and out. *[Pause.]*

Moving your awareness to just inside the nostrils, feeling the air passing in and out, warm and cool, dry and moist, in and out. *[Pause.]*

Moving your awareness to the tip of your nose, feeling whatever sensations are there. Your mind is like a microscope, focusing in on the smallest of sensations, finding the atoms of sensation.

For the remaining few minutes, we will stay with the sensations at the tip of the nose, allowing the breath to be natural, not forcing it, very soft, very gentle, very light, very quiet. *[Pause.]*

[Most of the children will be completely absorbed for at least five to ten minutes. Some of the children will naturally break their attention and begin looking around. For those with their eyes open, you can just smile and indicate they should keep silent (finger to lips sign) which will reassure them that they're not in trouble but should respect the others. When a critical mass of children have broken their concentration, close the meditation, as follows:]

Keeping the eyes closed, bring your attention to the palms of your hands, feeling them resting on your knees. Slowly lift your hands and feel the movement as you bring your hands up and then palms together in front of your chest, feeling all the sensations as we did before. *[Students will end up doing the palms-together movement much more slowly than they did earlier in the class, and this serves as a nice point of comparison. Allow the students to take their time.]* And now bring your hands back to your knees. Open your eyes to look at the floor just in front of you. Take a nice deep breath. And now open your eyes all the way. *[Give the students a big smile and look around the room. Teacher should stay quiet and relaxed, mirroring the energy of the room.]* Good job, everyone. Believe it or not, that was a ten-minute meditation. As we noted before, the quality of time changes when we're deeply attentive to the present moment.

Short Talk

While the students are in this quiet space is a time for you to say a few words about meditation. Your voice should stay soft, and you can slowly shift the energy of your speech as the students become wigglier and come out of their meditative space.

While we're in this quiet moment together, I just want you to notice how you feel. Does your mind feel like it has a little more space, like we've cleared out a bit of clutter? Do you feel more relaxed? Judging by your smiles, I can see that [some of] you do. And if you don't feel relaxed, that's okay too. Sometimes when we meditate we might actually feel a little worse. This is because we've gone from being numb to being more aware, and sometimes we're aware that we're not feeling quite right. Meditation is actually not about trying to feel good: it's about becoming aware of experience, whether it's pleasant, unpleasant, or neutral.

Meditation is also not about spacing out. It's not about going into a fantasy world. It's just the opposite. It's about connecting to our present moment experience and to ourselves in a very deep way. All the activities we have done have been about training our mind to focus on what's going on in the present moment. The wonderful thing about the present moment is that it is the least stressful moment to be in. Most of our thinking tends to be based in the past, remembering things, or based in the future, planning. Both the past and the future tend to cause us anxiety or stir up more thoughts. But the present moment is just what it is, and our mind, when really present, is unable to worry or judge. So it gives us a moment of rest.

But why do we focus on the breath? Breathing is a very special part of our being because the breath is a link between our body and our mind. In fact, our breathing often reflects our state of mind. When you are afraid, your breathing becomes short and tight and resides in the chest area. When you get surprised, you will take a quick, sharp breath into your throat area. But, get this: you can use your breath to control your state of mind. Let's do an experiment. I'd like everyone to put one hand on the belly and one hand on the chest. Now take a slow breath in, first letting the belly-hand rise and then draw air up into the chest, letting your chest-hand rise. Good. Now slowly breathe out, letting the chest-hand fall and then letting your belly-hand fall. Notice what your mind feels like: calm, relaxed, unworried. That's why when kids get mad a teacher might say, "Slow down, I want you to take three deep breaths." It really works: three deep breaths will calm our mind down.

And this is one reason that in meditation we use the breath as an anchor for our attention. We can place our attention on anything: on sound, on the taste of a raisin, on the body. But paying attention to the breath has an incredibly deep effect on the mind, giving it calmness and clarity. The next time you feel stressed out before a test, or angry at your parents, or frustrated with a sibling, try taking a deep breath. See if you feel calmer and clearer about how you want to respond to the situation.

While focusing on the breath has this special quality, it's also true that we can be mindful of anything. You don't have to sit on a cushion to practice mindfulness meditation. How so? Well, think about it. We were mindful of sounds at the beginning of this class. If you're walking from one place to another, try listening for how many sounds you can hear. We were mindful of a raisin after that. Imagine eating an entire meal mindfully! Believe it or not, that too is meditation. You can be mindful of walking. Walking meditation. In fact, this is the whole point of meditation: to be present and fully aware of yourself and all that is around you. To be mindful, to be engaged. But I also encourage you to dedicate some time to doing meditation formally in a quiet space. It helps train the mind so that when you go out into the world you have some capacity to pay attention. Try just doing five minutes a day, maybe in the morning before your mind gets too busy.

So let's review what we learned in this meditation class. Meditation is a practice that can help you decrease worry, stress, and anxiety and increase peacefulness, happiness, and a sense of well-being. Being mindful of what you are experiencing helps you enjoy that moment more. Meditation helps us be aware of our thoughts and emotions and helps us get to know ourselves better. Meditation increases our ability to pay attention, so naturally we will be better at sports, art, music, and studying. Meditation can be done anytime, anywhere.

But please don't feel pressured to do meditation. I am just offering this to you as a skill that you can draw upon in the future. Just as we learn how to use a pencil, ride a bike, or throw a ball, you can think of mindfulness meditation as a skill for dealing with things on the inside. So, when the time comes that you need a way to let go of stress or anxiety or you want to feel peaceful inside, then know that you now have the skill of mindfulness meditation at hand.

Mindfulness in Everyday Life: Homework Assignment

If you want to improve your ability to be mindful, then I recommend practicing mindfulness meditation during the times when you're bored or waiting for something. Let's say you're in the car, waiting for someone to put gas in the car. What do some of us do? Take out a cell phone and make a call, or perhaps send a little message to a friend? Maybe turn on the radio and fiddle around with it? Basically, most of us will do anything except sit there and be quiet, being present with our immediate environment. We crave stimulation and hate boredom. But here is a perfect opportunity to try something different. While you're waiting, close your eyes and play a game of discovering how many sounds you can hear. Can you hear the gurgle of the gas going into the car? The beeping of the machine when the credit card is approved? The receipt being printed?

So, here's your homework: find one activity that you do every day and use that moment to be fully mindful of what's going on. Maybe it's putting on your socks. You can put on your socks with total attention to the feeling of cloth against your skin, the pressure, your fingers, your toenails scraping the inside, and so on. Try noticing one new thing each day for a week. I'd like to go around the room and ask you what you will do for the next week as a mindfulness exercise.

Closing with Loving Kindness

We'll end with one last short activity. I'd like you to think about something you own that you really care about. Maybe it's your favorite pair of pants, or a baseball mitt, or a book you've read many times.

Now if I were to ask you to describe that thing to me, you'd be able to tell me every single last detail about it, right? For example, these pants I'm wearing. These are my favorite pair. I can tell you about the small threads here where a dog put his paws and ripped a little. The tiny little pen mark that I can't seem to wash out.

The point is that the things we love and care about we pay attention to. And very often, the things we pay attention to we come to love. For example, in my grandmother's house there's a painting that I used to think was pretty ugly. Well, I've had to pass that painting by for about the last ten years and because I've seen it so much, I actually have a little bit of affection for that painting. So love and attention are two sides to the same coin.

This morning, we've done a lot with our attention, learning about it, making it stronger. Now we'll close with just a little bit of love, the other side of the coin. Close your eyes and bring your attention inside yourself. Settling in to a comfortable, relaxed position. It's okay to lie down again if you prefer. Just make yourself very comfortable.

We're going to repeat three phrases silently in our minds.
May I be happy.
May I be peaceful.
May I be safe and protected.
[*Note: there are other classic phrases the teacher can draw from:*
   May I take care of myself easily.
   May I accept myself for all that/who I am.
   May I be free from suffering.
   May I have ease of well-being.
   May I be free from inner and outer harm.]
Teacher repeats these three phrases at least 3-4 times. It can be helpful to add some guidance, such as:
   "I truly and sincerely wish: May I be happy…."
   "With all my heart, I wish: May I be happy…"
   "With all my good intentions, I hope that: May I be happy…"
   "Remembering that I am a good person, full of kindness, intelligence, humor, generosity, I wish for myself: May I be happy…"

Now, without opening your eyes, think of the person to your right. "Person to my right, whether I know you well or whether I know you only a little, I truly and sincerely wish for you, May you be happy. May

you be peaceful. May you be free from harm. Just as I wish for myself these things, I wish for you….May you be…"
[Do 3-4 times.]
Now, without opening your eyes, think of the person to your left.
"Person to my left, whether I know you well …"
[Do 3-4 times.]
Now thinking of our teachers here with us today, with all the care and attention they give us, "Dear teacher, I wish you for you,…."
"Thinking of all our classmates here in this room…." *[Phrase can change to "May we all be happy."]*
Finally, let's think about the whole school. Everyone here having joys and sorrows, challenges and successes. The younger and older children who come here, the dedicated and kind teachers, the people who make our food and feed us, the janitors who clean the hallways and shoveled the snow today, the secretaries, the administrators, everyone in our whole school, who are all good people, let us wish for everyone, "May we all be happy…."
[When finished, let there be some silence.]
Okay, open your eyes and come into a sitting position. Wonderful, very good everyone.
[And then the teacher can close with:]
You have been such a great group to work with. Thank you for your wholehearted effort. I truly wish for each of you here, May you be happy… [something of a final word from the teacher, giving loving kindness to the children].

Notes for the Teacher

Demonstrating: For true beginners, I found that the more the teacher demonstrates, the better the results. For example, when demonstrating the mindfulness of palms coming together activity, the kinds of experiences you note will be a model for the students:

    Warmth of palms on the knees
    Contraction of biceps
    Cool air under the palms
    Inevitably, these will be the points that the students list when they do it. But if you are more detailed in your noting, students will be more creatively detailed in theirs:
    As my fingers separate, feeling the moisture between them cool off
    The twitching of my left, fourth finger
    A ripple of muscle contraction in my shoulder

Still, students will need encouragement to discover their own experiences, to see if they can come up with something unique that you haven't said.

Discipline: If a student is out of line, giggly or slouchy or keeps their eyes open a lot, that's *okay*. In my experience, because of the nature of these activities, scolding or sternness is not appropriate. Students open their eyes perhaps because they're uncomfortable. In that case, just smiling at them reassures them that they're safe with you. Or, I found that just placing my hand on the student's shoulder helps calm them down.

Support teacher: If you have more than twelve students who are teenagers or younger, I recommend including one support teacher for each eight to twelve more students. The support teacher is there to help with behavioral issues that might arise and to ground the energy of the room.

About you, as the teacher:

- *Be calm, loving, positive, and energetic.* The most critical element of teaching meditation is presence and conduct. Children will watch to see whether the teacher embodies meditative qualities. Teachers should have good posture and project presence, authority, and warmth from the belly.

- *Be yourself.* Young people are drawn to meditation because they believe it offers them the opportunity to experience something real and authentic. Children will appreciate being able to connect to the teacher in his or her authenticity.

- *Practice meditation.* To speak intimately and genuinely about meditation, the teacher needs to have practiced, and continue to practice, meditation.

- *Don't underestimate:* Teachers often report that they are surprised not only by the children's ability to pick up meditation quickly but also by their astute observations and deep experiences. Children will feel the teacher respects their capacity to meditate if the teacher quietly sets high expectations.

- *Environment:* If possible, hold the class in a place that has a minimum of outside distraction (such as a room without windows that look out on a busy sidewalk) and noise (white noise like traffic is fine, but nearby audible conversations are distracting). Meditation mats or even carpet remnants can make kids feel that they have a dedicated sitting spot of their own. Ceremonial or beautiful objects, such as a vase of flowers, candles, or even a Buddha statue in a meditative pose (not recommended for public school spaces, though) also help create a special setting.

- *Parent involvement:* If it is possible to have parents join the class, do! There are many advantages: it puts the parents on the same level as the children, since all are students learning something new. The children will watch their parents for modeling and possibly follow their example. It is beneficial for the parents to learn meditation. And the parents will be able to support and encourage mindfulness in the home for all family members.

Beanie Baby Meditation

Mary Scattergood

In my sixteen years of teaching I have become keenly aware of the pressures and demands that confront young children today. Even in a loving, nurturing and community-based Quaker school such as Friends School Haverford, where I teach, students experience a hurried lifestyle very different from the one I knew growing up. Children's schedules are so full that they have little time for play and relaxation; they become frazzled and out of sync. Their fast-paced lives resemble those of the adults. There is little time to wonder, to be in nature, to play games of make-believe. Their inner lives, potentially rich places for imaginative and inventive activity, are withering from lack of engagement in just being a child and experiencing childhood in a more natural state.

In my own childhood, I remember delighting in afternoons of endless free play with neighborhood children. There was often a parent at home so that we moved freely and safely between homes, sharing suppers together or being read to by a grandmother. I have memories of climbing magnolia trees, inventing outdoor plays, and stealing sugar lumps from my grandmother's pantry. We had time to notice, to wonder, and to just be with our surroundings. Today there is little time for children to breathe, admire a flower, enjoy a sunset, or catch a firefly. The sacred moments of childhood are at risk of disappearing.

Last summer, looking for a way to develop further clarity of mind, I joined a meditation group to study and practice meditation regularly. As I my practice developed, I found meditation a useful tool for being present in full, clear awareness from moment to moment in a more skillful way. The sense of urgency, reactivity, and hurrying through my day began to shift. I became conscious of the importance of listening, observing, and connecting with others and my surroundings with mindfulness and authenticity. In so doing my life became less stressful, and I became aware of the preciousness of life and how short a time we have on this earth. I began to think about my teaching practice in a different light. I knew that by serving myself, in effect, I could better serve others. I wanted to communicate this new way of being with my students and lead them to create a community where reflection, stress reduction, and mindfulness could be an integral part of classroom life.

Our students are familiar with moments of silence because of their experience in Quaker Meeting. As my second-graders discussed their experience of Meeting for Worship, I led into a discussion about meditation. Some children were familiar with the term. Several students showed me the lotus pose and made humming noises meant to resemble mantras. I acknowledged their poses and mantras and explained that I would like to try an experiment with them. Could each of them watch their breath go in (we call that inhalation) and follow it down into an exhalation. I demonstrated, placing my hands on my belly, carefully executing each inhalation and exhalation. On each inhalation I counted one and on each exhalation I counted two. Soon everyone was following along, mostly exaggerating his or her breaths, giggling, and becoming unglued and very silly. This is par for the course, I thought, for second-graders. I'll have to come up with something more developmentally friendly. I knew that my approach to mindfulness training would have to engage their interest a well as their developmental readiness for a practice.

Over time, I created an activity that we call "Beanie Baby Meditation." Although I'm not a proponent of using commercial playthings as a way of getting children's attention, the fact is that some do. My acceptance and respect for their interest in these stuffed animals allowed me to be playful while teaching mindfulness at the same time. The Beanie Babies became the tool for them to "Tune In." Here's how it began.

> The sound of the gong resonates as second-graders gather on the rug for morning circle. "Did you all remember to bring your Beanie Babies today?" I ask. A chorus of joyful voices and laughter fill the classroom.
>
> "I brought George, my cat Beanie," says John. "What's the name of your Beanie, Tanisha?"
>
> "She's called Piggy—because she's a pig, of course!"
>
> Students squirm and wiggle as they introduce their small stuffed animals to each other.
>
> "Do you remember how we've been counting our breaths, our inhalations, and our exhalations with our eyes closed and our hands on our bellies?" I inquire.
>
> "Yes," says Ryan. "That's called meditation."

"It's when we get real quiet inside, kind of like Meeting for Worship," suggests Sarah.

"That's right, Sarah," I say. "We feel our bellies go out on breath one, and in on breath two. In and out, in and out..."

"We know that, Ms. Scat," interrupts Philip. "How come we got to bring our Beanie Babies to circle?"

"Philip," I answer, catching his gaze, "Today we're going to practice Beanie Baby meditation."

"Yeah...whoopee!" There are giggles and squeals of delight from my ten animated students.

"Before we begin," I instruct in my quietest voice, "find a comfortable resting spot on the floor. Lie down and place your Beanie on your belly. Gently close your eyes and place your arms by your side." Gradually, the mood shifts as the children and their stuffed pets settle into silence. At the sound of the gong, we breathe in on the count of one, and out on the count of two.

As the gong rings, I say, "Feel your Beanie rise on the in-breath and lower on the out-breath. Follow my counts...one...two...three." I continue on to ten. The room is magically still, with almost no sound except the rustle of leaves outside the classroom window. For this brief moment my young students are utterly focused.

"When you're ready," I whisper, "very slowly and carefully turn your body to one side and gently sit up. Place your Beanie in the middle of the circle and remain silent."

Ten pairs of eye gaze up at me. We are quiet and relaxed, ready to start the school day. It works!

Since that day, we have built Beanie Baby meditation into our weekly schedule. Another small practice that I incorporate throughout the day is a "pause break" whenever I see a need for it. I ring the gong and they know to come to their seats and place their heads on their desks. We watch our breathing while I count in-breath one, and out-breath two for a round of ten. These refreshment breaks help settle restless bodies and minds and give us a chance to refocus with more clarity on the previous activity or prepare for the next activity.

I observe that these quieting, reflective activities assist children in reaching a feeling of relaxation and calm, and help increase concentration and focus. If schools provide students with intentional practices of "tuning in," we potentially create an educational environment that deepens a child's appreciation for herself and others, and in a larger sense, we open a window onto the world.

Muscles, Pebbles, and Good Will

Irene McHenry

This essay presents three mindfulness activities that are easy to teach and to learn, well received by others, and effective in the classroom and in therapeutic settings with young children, adolescents, and adults. They are mind as a muscle, pebble practice, and good will practice. These practices develop the natural and unique human capacity to deepen and strengthen awareness, to hone the skill of concentration, to sharpen emotional health, and to strengthen the mind-body system's access to a state of well-being that is simultaneously relaxed and alert. Enhanced awareness can lead to deeper satisfaction with learning and with living, and the practice of breath concentration gives everyone a useful, handy, readily available tool for use in any situation of stress, overwhelm, anxiety, and that dreaded adolescent state of mind— boredom.

Mind as a Muscle

One major benefit of using mindfulness practices routinely in the academic classroom is that the students' capacity to concentrate is enhanced. A brief daily practice of being with the experience of the breath can build not only relaxation skills but also the ability to focus attention over longer periods of time. I have used this "Mind as a Muscle" activity successfully with seventh-grade students in a course that meets daily at the William Penn Charter School as well as in one-time presentations as a guest teacher in grades eight through twelve.

The Theory

Beginning with an invitation to students (or clients) to think about their own minds and how the mind works and develops, I introduce the concept that the mind is different from and more expansive than the brain. The brain is part of the exquisite human nervous system that picks up information from all of our sensory experience and processes it, whereas the mind can be aware of the brain's processing while it happens, while simultaneously being aware of all external and internal sensations and all past and present experience. This idea kindles rich and fruitful discussion, especially among adolescents.

The next concept is that the mind, like any muscle, can be strengthened through routine practice, just as regular physical exercise enhances the ability to play a sport, just as regular practice on an instrument leads to strengthened ability to play and perform. Students are eager to provide detailed examples of their "practice" disciplines in sports, music, and theatre and to describe the muscle-building process in terms of the daily and weekly routines and the particular muscles and skills developed.

We talk about using the mind muscle to support all human activities, such as day-to-day living and problem-solving, development of any skill, attending to relationships with others. I introduce the idea that one of the major uses of the mind muscle is for centering in a relaxed and focused way, a way of *being* while doing any activity. We talk about centering as a countercultural notion—a challenge for us, given the pace and style of life in our culture, where we are constantly bombarded in our environments with stimulation to all of our senses. We brainstorm the sources of constant stimulation in our culture—audio, visual, and kinesthetic. Then, we talk about the idea of silence. Where do we have times in our daily life to stop activity and be silent? We reflect on times and places where students have experienced moments of silence in their lives.

Then I invite the students to experiment with an activity of "centering" as a way of strengthening the muscle of the mind by enhancing its ability to observe, focus, concentrate, and learn, all at the same time.

The Practice

After the introductory conversation, which may take place all at one time or over several meetings, I invite the students to experiment with an activity to develop the muscle of the mind. This experiment involves sitting in a centered posture with feet flat on the floor, the "sit bones" relaxed and solid on the chair, the spine rising upright naturally from the sit bones, the body relaxed. I use the image of a tree for this posture. The soles of the feet and the sit bones are like the roots of the tree, holding the ground, supporting the weight. The spine is like the trunk of the tree, rising up naturally toward the sky. The shoulders and arms are like the limbs of the tree, resting gracefully and without effort. I suggest closing the eyes for this experiment in order to close off a major source of stimulation, external images. If closing the eyes is uncomfortable, then narrowing the focus of the eyes toward the floor at a forty-five degree angle with a focus on one spot may achieve the same purpose of eliminating the distraction of external images. A very thorough discussion of posture and preparing to do sitting meditation in general can be found in Jon Kabat-Zinn's book, *Wherever You Go, There You Are.*

The experiment begins with the invitation to focus the muscle of the mind on the experience of breathing for thirty seconds. The goal is not to do anything with the breath, just notice the breath moving in and out of the body without effort, and notice the accompanying sensations of the breath's natural, changing movement. I use a small chime to indicate the beginning and the end of the thirty seconds. Midpoint in this brief time period, I remind students to pay attention to the experience of breathing in and the experience of breathing out. After the experiment, I ask students what they noticed: What was easy? What was challenging? What was comfortable? What was uncomfortable? What sounds did they notice in the background? What thoughts (image thoughts and word thoughts), worries, feelings, and sensations did they notice while focusing their minds on their breathing? Were these thoughts or feelings distracting or did they stay in the background with the focus on the breath staying in the foreground?

I ask if they think they could do this experiment again, but for one minute rather than thirty seconds. I suggest keeping an awareness of sensations other than the breath (sounds, thoughts, images, body sensations, emotional feelings) in the background while keeping the main focus of the awareness on the breath. I use the metaphor of a flashlight shining a beam of light on the breathing experience. Again, we begin and end the experiment with the chime. At the end of sixty seconds, I again ask what they noticed and encourage description rather than evaluation. I am careful to validate each experience; one is not better than another. We talk about how this experiment will likely be a different experience every time they try it, and I encourage them to try it frequently during the day, such as at the beginning of each new class.

When done daily in a class, we experiment for one week by starting each class with the muscle-mind centering practice. We try different amounts of time each day: thirty seconds, sixty seconds, two minutes. Each time, I ask students what they notice during the experiment, making space for acceptance of all observations without judgment. Frequently, and at first to my surprise, the seventh-grade boys, with a healthy, competitive "can-do" spirit, wanted to increase the time each day. I remind students that this is not a competition; this is an exploration. I invite students to try the centering practice at other times during the day and to let me know what they are noticing. Seventh-graders have described feeling more calm before tests, less irritable in class, less anxious before a competitive sports event, and looking forward to settling into class in this way. If I ever forget to begin class with the chime and the centering, they are quick to remind me.

Pebble Practice

Four pebbles; four breaths; four phrases to guide the breath.

I have used this simple focusing activity with young children, preschool through elementary age. I have also adapted it for teachers and school administrators and for executives in non-profit organizations to use for stress relief and refreshment. Teachers can easily adapt this activity to be developmentally appropriate for the age of the children they teach. The concepts and actual phrases are adapted from the work of Thich Nhat Hanh.

Pebble practice helps students learn the skill of calm centering and helps them develop concentration through focusing on the breath. While calming the mind and giving the body a systematic routine, students develop the skill of concentration and at the same time, experience relaxation. This result creates a perfect context in the mind-body system for learning: the alert, relaxed mind.

Pebble practice is a sound, developmental activity for the brain and for sensory-motor integration, as it involves physically crossing the midline of the body. It also develops coordination and awareness of the body in space as well as practice with right-left directions. In preparing for pebble practice, teachers can develop language-based activities introducing the words for the four phrases that are used in the exercise: in-out, deep-slow, calm-ease, here-now. One activity could be learning about opposites (such as in-out, deep-shallow, calm-stormy, ease-difficulty). Other activities might include brainstorming similarities to each word, acting out each word, and talking about concrete examples of the experience of each word.

Another introductory activity before experimenting with pebble practice can be exploring the physiology of the breath. How does it work? Where does it come from? How does it work when we are sleeping? When we are awake? Where is it most easy to notice that the breath is moving through the body? The students can be invited to try noticing the movement of the breath in the nose, the throat, the chest, the belly. What does it feel like to hold the breath? To release it? What does the breath do for the body and the brain?

Let the students know that the focus on the breath can be used for calming and centering at any time, such as settling down after recess, getting centered before a reading activity, getting centered to do homework, or calming down at any time of frustration or anxiety.

Materials:

1. Enough pebbles (or other small natural objects, such as twigs, sea shells), so that each student can use four of the small objects. Gathering the natural objects out-of-doors can be a special activity in itself. Later, children can cut squares of fabric and stitch small bags for safekeeping of their pebbles or twigs.

2. Small cards, one for each student, with the four phrases printed on them. For young children, print the phrases on chart paper and review the words as a language-building activity.

3. A small chime.

The phrases:

(On the in-breath)   *(On the out-breath)*
in. . . . . out
deep . . . . slow
calm . . . . ease
here . . . . now

A. Breathing as a solo practice

- Introduce the activity with a discussion of how the mind works and teach the idea of calm, relaxed attention as a core skill for learning anything.

- Invite the students to sit in a circle cross-legged on the floor. Alternatively, children could sit at tables or desks.

- Bring a large quantity of pebbles (lovely, polished small pebbles are available in craft shops), and invite each student to take four pebbles from a bowl that is passed around. Instruct students to place the pebbles at their right sides. (Alternatively, students can explore in the outside world and discover four pebbles that they bring into the classroom.)

- Model and practice a portion of the activity together before doing the complete activity.

- When the directions and practice session have been completed with eyes open, invite students to close their eyes and try moving the pebbles by touch. Using a chime, indicate that the sound of the chime invites them to close their eyes and the second sounding of the chime, invites them to open their eyes.

- For moving the pebbles, invite the children to move each pebble on one complete breath. Take one pebble in the right hand from the right side of the body and while moving the arm in an arc toward the left side of the body, inhale. Then, while exhaling and keeping the pebble in the right hand, place the pebble down at the left side of the body (demonstrate). To guide the movement and the breath, say a word for each in-breath and a different word for each out-breath (in/out, deep/slow, calm/ease, here/now).

- Say the first word to indicate the beginning of the inhalation, which last to the midpoint of the arc, then speak the second word of the phrase for the exhalation.

- When the four phrases have been completed and the four pebbles moved to the left side, repeat the activity, if desired, with moving the pebbles, one on each breath, back to the right side. (The activity can be further repeated by doing one complete round with the right hand and one complete round with the left hand.)

- Throughout the demonstration, and at the end of the whole activity, ask the children what they notice about their experience. Validate each observation. Refrain from making evaluative remarks.

- Invite the children to use their pebbles on their own whenever they wish to calm down, refresh, and refocus.

B. Breathing as a group practice

The group activity develops relational awareness of being a member of a group. It is a wonderful community activity emphasizing cooperation and the concept of interdependence.

- Invite students to be seated on the floor in a circle.

- Ask students to choose only one of their four pebbles for this activity. Invite them to really get to know the pebble by size, shape, color, feel.

- Invite the students to place the pebble on the floor or on the desk at the right side of their bodies.

- Use the same phrases and movement as with the solo activity above. However, instruct the students that each time they complete the arc by placing the pebble at their left side, the person to their left will be picking up that pebble for the next phrase's in-breath.

- Then, with the second and each subsequent phrase, each student reaches for the pebble on her right, which has been placed there by the person to her right.

- Continue the activity until the starting pebble comes back to its starting person. (If you as the teacher, participate in the circle, then you will know when your special pebble returns.)

- Open and close the activity with the sound of the bell.

- Ask the children what they noticed or experienced.

Pebble Practice After-Thoughts

A school guidance counselor emailed a message to me after a mindfulness workshop saying that two days after she arrived back at work, her school principal had a heart attack and died during the night. She was called early in the morning and told to come to school as quickly as possible to be available for the students and teachers. While driving to school in shock and wondering how she could work with others while she was experiencing deep grief, she remembered the four phrases from pebble practice used to support the breath and calm the body-mind system. She used the phrases with her breath during the ten-minute drive to school. She said that by the time she arrived, she felt quite calm, relaxed and alert, and was able to focus on her work for the day supporting others in the school community.

Another school guidance counselor reported that she had the four phrases printed on wallet-sized cards and gave them to the teenagers in her weekly "chat" groups. She taught them the simple practice of the breath. Many of her students have told her that they carry the cards in their wallets and use this practice often to calm down when they are feeling overwhelmed with strong emotions.

In using this practice with heads of schools and with administrators of non-profit organizations, we use four polished pebbles in a small bowl, sized just right to sit on a desk. I recommend using the pebble practice many times throughout the busy workday. It only takes a moment to focus on the breath, with the aid of moving the pebbles, in order to feel refreshed and centered for continuing with work.

Practicing Good Will

In the classroom and in group work with adults, I have found that teaching a mindfulness practice called "good will" (traditionally known as loving kindness meditation or metta) provides a valuable pathway to increase awareness of self and of others in a positive context. By way of introduction, I say that practicing good will strengthens and expands our ordinary human love-ability.

The goal of the practice is to intentionally produce positive thoughts that evoke feelings of love and good will toward oneself and toward others. This "good will" practice can reduce stress, ease frustration, increase the mind's capacity to embrace the full reality of "what is," and create an experience of a calm, centered state of being.

The practice uses a structured series of phrases that convey intentions of good will. The precise wording of the phrases and the precise order of the phrases is not as important as the intention. The practice and phrases that I commonly use with students and teachers are from *Beginning Mindfulness: Learning the Way of Awareness,* by Andrew Weiss. There are five cycles of intention, beginning with directing good will toward the self, then extending good will toward an acquaintance or a stranger, then to a person you know and like, then to a person you love dearly, and finally, to a person you despise or fear.

The leader speaks each phrase aloud slowly, so that one full inhalation and exhalation can take place on one phrase. Then, the leader can pause and instruct the group to say the phrase silently to themselves while continuing to focus on the breath. Continue with each phrase, giving ample time to savor the affirmation and the breath.

May I be well and happy.
May I be strong, confident, and peaceful.
May I have ease and well-being.

The phrases are changed to "May you ..." for the remaining four cycles (extending good will toward an acquaintance or a stranger, then to a person you know and like, then to a person you love dearly, and finally, to a person you despise or fear.)

May you be well and happy.
May you be strong, confident, and peaceful.
May you have ease and well-being.

I encourage teachers to feel free to be creative in adapting this good will practice after becoming familiar with it. For example, you may repeat each single phrase or each sequence of phrases several times, or you may focus just on saying one of the phrases over and over. You may also create your own words to convey your intentions of love and good will. Invite students to develop one or more affirmative phrases for the practice, and use the students' words for daily or weekly variety.

A rich discussion can be developed from this practice about the meaning of happiness. What does it take to be happy? Are there degrees of happiness? How do we know when we are in a state of happiness? When do we naturally feel happy? Take advantage of a teachable moment in the discussion to provide the traditional Buddhist meaning of the concept of happiness in this meditation: "happy" indicates the concept of contentment without conditions, without desiring or avoiding, without wanting anything to be different than it is. This lifts the conversation to a new level of inquiry. Is happiness possible without conditions? What is unconditional love? What does it mean to have good will toward self and others?

Learning Silence and Reflection Through the Body: Yoga Class

Barry Blumenfeld

The bell rings and students trickle into the narrow dance studio. They chat about their day as they change out of their clothes into something loose and comfortable. They grab a yoga mat, perhaps a blanket, too, and gravitate to what has become their usual spot. There are ninth-graders clustered together toward the back; the seniors all rush to be in the front row. Soon the room is filled, and stragglers squeeze in and unroll their mats as I take a seat on the floor. Some students are still chatting while others lay on their mats with their eyes closed. I ask the students to turn their awareness to their breathing: Is it deep? Shallow? Fast? Slow? Once the room has come to a full stillness, together we breathe a deep inhalation and chant the sound "Om"—our individual sounds forming one vibration and in many ways marking the moment we all say, "We are here, now."

The very first class of each semester I teach students the word "Om" from the yoga philosophy of sound. There are many different ideas about the meaning of "Om." I tell students that, in general, "Om" is considered to be the sound of the vibration of creation. I tell them that if nothing else, by "Om"-ing together, we tune in to each other, creating a community unified in sound, intention, and the present moment.

I teach yoga at Friends Seminary School in Manhattan, and I strive to make every class an expression of mindful stillness, activity, learning, and relationships. A goal of each class is to teach students skills for becoming grounded in the present moment and bringing consciousness to the present circumstance. The ever-confident juniors and seniors who have taken yoga with me before join in the class discussion, challenging the ideas or affirming them, connecting them to lessons they have learned in other classes.

We often discuss compassion as a theme, and during our annual "Peace Week" we practice an affirmation that comes from a classical form of meditation called metta or loving kindness. We have used the following affirmations in silent meditation:

May I feel protected and safe.
May I feel contented and pleased.
May my physical body bring me strength.
May my life unfold smoothly, with ease.

Then we use these same affirmations, focusing them on people we love, people we like, people we are indifferent about, and people we dislike.

Next, we practice a variety of yogic breathing techniques. Developing an awareness of the breath gives students a tool to be calmly present in a stressful situation. In yoga the breath work is called pranayama, which translates to "expansion of the life force," so not only are we being present, we are increasing our vitality.

Then, as the students move into the yoga postures, I continually remind them that the true practice is not about getting the postures "right," but practicing how to breathe into a physical pose while still remaining conscious and focused on the breath. By doing this, they are training themselves to be centered. I encourage them not to judge themselves in a pose, rather to accept themselves with full awareness of their bodies in space. Students learn to balance an intense physical practice with deep relaxation through the breath. We complete the postures with the "corpse pose." It's not a big surprise that this is the students' favorite pose, as it involves lying on their backs, closing their eyes and completely relaxing into the present moment and letting the relaxation soak in deeply.

Because they are at a Friends school that regularly has Meeting for Worship, the practices of silence and reflective awareness are not foreign concepts to our students. Other teachers use centering practices and meditation in their classrooms. One math teacher begins each class by saying, "OK—let's settle" and then rings a chime. The students sit and listen to the chime, settle and relax, without doing anything else as the chime dies down, then they begin with homework review. The teacher introduces the chime in the beginning of the year as an auditory division between the world outside and the space inside as a math class. The chime opening is an opportunity to let go of the baggage that the students accumulate during the day so that they are more available to be present in the moment, ready to learn.

Yoga seems to be a natural fit for our physical education curriculum, which honors the many different types of physical abilities of our students. A large number of students play a sport for their PE requirement, but for those who do not consider themselves athletes we added options such as fitness, fencing, tap dancing, and modern dance. Yoga was added as a physical education option five years ago to diversify the program further. The combination of stretching and strengthening, which develop awareness of the breath and mindfulness of the body, along with a structure that allows students to set their own level of challenge, made it ideal for our program. From the first semester it was offered, the response was overwhelming. The first class filled up quickly, so a second section was added. Two sections of two classes a week continue to be offered.

The students love yoga, and members of all upper school grade levels, 9-12, seek to join the classes. Usually there are 12 to 15 students in a section of yoga, but some who are not enrolled stop by just to take a class when they are free. Students sit down on their mats, heave a heavy sigh, and exclaim how happy they are to be in class. One student told me that at the beginning of class she is usually tired and when she focuses on her breath she worries because she finds it shallow. At the end of class, however, she is energized, has no trouble sitting still in silence, and enjoys easy, deep breaths.

I close all of my yoga classes by bringing the practice back to silence, and then the students and I chant the Sanskrit word *Shanti*, which means peace. After chanting *Shanti* three times, we bow and I recite my wish for them: "May there peace in your thoughts, peace in your words, peace in your heart, and peace in all your day. *Namaste.*" *Namaste* can be translated as "The light in me honors the light in you." The students, now focused, calm, and relaxed, respond, "*Namaste.*"

Exploring Mindfulness
with Elementary School Students

Judy Belasco

Eight years ago I attended a mindfulness workshop with Richard Brady and Irene McHenry. I enjoyed learning walking meditation and eating meditation as well as participating in the group experiences. The retreat renewed my long-time desire to share centering tools with my students in the art classes I teach to grades one through five at Germantown Friends School, a Quaker school in Philadelphia. An inspiration to use a Tibetan singing bowl to begin my classes came to me. Irene encouraged me to try it, and suggested using simple, direct language without any religious references.

Soon after the retreat, I went to a local Tibetan store to get a singing bowl. The shopkeeper graciously showed me how to move the wooden stick around the outside of the bowl to allow the polyphonic sounds to emerge. He explained that the bowls were made from seven metals, then he left me alone to try bowl after bowl. I was eventually drawn to an ancient-looking, unpolished and slightly rusty bowl.

I took the bowl to school. For several years I had been using a high-pitched chime to begin my classes, so the change to the bowl was very easy. The students liked it immediately. During the first few months, we gradually formulated how we would use the bowl, creating our own ritual. Our love of doing it has made it a revered practice that works the same way each time.

The students arrive in the art room and sit around a large table. After the initial greeting and gathering I ask the students, "Are you ready?" I unwrap the sounding stick from its special piece of purple rice paper and I say very softly, "Please close your eyes gently." This instruction is very deliberate, as it helps them to relax their facial muscles. I wait for real silence. I sound the bowl with a little tap to wake it up and allow a little more silence before I actually begin. As I move the stick slowly around the bowl, the sound emanating from it changes from barely audible to filling the whole room with its hum. As I lift the stick away, a ringing sound adds into the hum, and we listen intently as the polyphonic sounds fall slowly away into a rich and full silence. I ask the students to indicate when they no longer hear the bowl by placing their hands under their chins. I glance around and end the experience with a cascade of very lightly tinkling chimes. They open their eyes. We all smile. We are together.

These steps of the bowl experience evolved over the course of several years. I knew that when I asked students to close their eyes it was to enable them to listen intently without visual stimuli. But not all students followed that request. I finally had the insight to ask students to close their eyes in order to generously allow everyone, including me, absolute privacy throughout the experience. I explained that no one wants a dozen people staring at them if they're the last one to put their hand under their chin. I also wanted to protect people who may have involuntary facial expressions. The request for privacy really resonates with the students and they respect, honor, and understand it.

When we emerge from the short, intense, deep meditation with the bowl we are all ready to listen. As a teacher I do not have to demand attention because we *are* attention. I can practically whisper directions for art.

Using the bowl is a privilege that I feel every time we do it. However, if I am not in a centered place when I sound the bell, it clangs harshly and I have to focus deeply and quickly to be in harmony again. Although it happens infrequently, I like to share my own distractibility with the students so they understand that this is an ongoing issue for all of us.

As my actual experience does not have special relevance, I generally share nothing about it, although sometimes I ask if they also heard a sound that I heard. Lately students have shared spontaneously out of a sense of wonder and awe. A student said recently as he emerged from the silence, "Everything looks so light." Another student commented, "I see blue dots everywhere." I simply smile and say, "Yes."

I recently introduced the scale of chimes to bring the experience of silence to a close. Next, I said that I was going to give them a question that does not have one specific answer, as some questions do not have an answer. I asked, "Why do we smile when we hear the chimes?" Although we all smiled, we have yet to discuss it; we enjoy the experience of wondering.

Recently, I asked several classes across the first to fifth grades to share with me what happened for them. I asked, "What is your feeling or experience when we do the bowl?" We went around in a circle and nearly everyone spoke. The most prevalent answers were that it makes them feel "calm, happy, relaxed, quiet, peaceful, good, concentrated, joyful, and cheerful." Other responses were more unusual:

I have a lot of energy and it calms me down.
I like the vibration.
I stop worrying about the past or future and focus on now.
It makes me feel in a safe place.
It makes me more aware of my surroundings.
It erases my mind and I see how nice the sound is.
It helps me to focus on whatever I am doing.
It makes me sad. My father died.
It makes me comfortable, settled down and on track.
I have a distant memory of being a baby.
It stops my hunger pains.
It makes me feel peaceful. That moment is my moment;
    no one can take it from me.
It helps me stop being silly and stop talking to friends.

After exploring this question with a few classes, I posed another: "If you see anything when your eyes are closed, what do you see?" The common and excited answer was, "Color." The colors ranged across the spectrum. I was surprised at the number of students who reported seeing colors. Some of the more elaborate answers:

I see sparkles like stars.
I see colorful butterflies.
I see whirls and swirls.
I see two silver lights, then a small light which explodes
    into a pool of color.
I feel like I am in heaven.
I see a parrot flying in a landscape.

After three years of sounding the bowl to begin all of my classes, I became interested in trying walking meditation with the students. Every other Thursday in our school, we have formal Meeting for Worship in the Friends Meetinghouse; on the alternate Thursdays we choose another venue for an informal Meeting for Worship. I decided to try walking meditation as an alternative Meeting for Worship with a second-grade class. Because it was winter, I thought it would be best to walk in the auditorium. When the class gathered, I started by reading some excerpts from Thich Nhat Hahn's book for children, *A Pebble in Your Pocket*. I then gave very brief instructions for coordinating breathing and steps while walking, and we began. As we walked, we paused periodically to listen when I sounded the bell.

After the period of walking meditation ended, we sat in silence for five minutes. To conclude, we shared our experiences, which ranged from feeling calm and peaceful to wondering if we were going to fall over. The idea was generally well received, so I extended a year-long offer to any class that wanted to try walking meditation during alternative meeting days.

Finally, a fifth-grade classroom teacher requested that I introduce sitting meditation, and I was happy to try. We used a dimly lit music room with a blue carpet and we sat cross-legged on the floor. I used a set of tinkling chimes for the centering sound.

I began the session by suggesting the purpose of meditation using Quaker terminology. I explained that we were setting the climate to connect to the Inner Light or to contact the Inner Teacher. I reminded the students that we all may have different ways of learning. Some people are comfortable with visual learning, others prefer auditory experiences, some like kinesthetic means, while still others resonate with feelings. I explained that different forms of meditation work in the same say. I said that we would do four short meditations using one method at a time to enter the interior domain. I suggested that the students may like one, two, or none of these experiences. I also shared that meditation is not really a time to think, although thinking naturally occurs.

I began with an auditory meditation because that is what we do together in art with the bowl. This time I introduced chanting as a means to still the mind and enter the inner space. Since we were chanting the word Om, I briefly explained its use and meaning in Eastern religions. "Om" is the primordial word according to ancient sages of India and has the power inherent in its sound to return us to a sense of inner oneness and peace. It is a tool to enter meditation. We then chanted together on one note but not in unison, allowing ourselves to breathe naturally as we chanted. We continued chanting for several minutes and then meditated silently for about five minutes. I end each meditation with the tinkling chimes because they very gently return our awareness to the room.

The second meditation I used is visual and very simple. I asked the students to close their eyes and just look at the field they saw there. I suggested that when thoughts intruded they come back to the field in front of their eyes. We meditated like this for five minutes.

The third meditation was kinesthetic; I guided them to watch their breath as it came in and out. If they needed help in "seeing" the breath I invited them to place their hands on their sides for a while to become more familiar with the movement. I asked them to return to their breath as needed to help them center during the meditation.

The fourth meditation focused awareness on an emotion; this is traditionally thought of as a devotional pathway. I led a very short guided meditation. I asked the students to visualize someone they loved a lot (a person or an animal) standing in their inner space and looking directly at them. I asked them to become as aware of the feeling of love as they were able. Then I suggested that they gradually let the loved one fade away, but retain the feeling of love and let that feeling glide them into meditation.

I often do variations on all of these meditations as I am led to, but this is the basic introduction to sitting meditation that I offer. The students help me to shape what works best for them because we always leave some time for sharing experiences at the end of each session.

The practices I draw on are the ancient paths of yoga and mindfulness training. I am grateful for the help, wisdom, and freshness of these practices. Teaching them is an evolving experiment in doing and learning from doing. To work with these varied and beautiful ways of helping all of us to center, to become aware, and to find calm in a noisy and distracted world is a great privilege. I hope that perhaps one small seed will blossom later in a student's life when it is most needed. To practice together is a joy, to increase awareness is a perfect complement to learning, and to focus deeply is truly satisfying. I am very happy that the students like it so much.

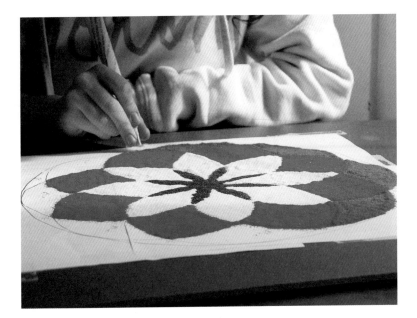

PART II
Quaker Practices
that Center in Mindfulness

Part II addresses mindfulness in the context of Quaker practices in
Friends school settings, especially the practice of Meeting for Worship.
The ideas shared can be easily adapted for use in any public or private
school setting toward the goal of developing core mindfulness skills for
learning: concentration, observation, relaxation, and emotional balance.
In secular educational settings, teachers can create simple names for
these practices, such as quiet time, centering time, settling in, or silent
meeting.

There are rich connections between mindfulness practices and Quaker
practices rooted in being in touch with the Spirit within oneself and
others. In this Part teachers explore these connections and describe
how they draw on them to help students enter more fully into Quaker

Meeting for Worship. Teachers also describe other Quaker practices that employ and cultivate mindfulness in students and in teachers.

Irene McHenry leads off Part II with an in-depth account of Meeting for Worship in Friends schools and descriptions of activities that "develop reflection, concentration, awareness, observation and centered relaxation" to help students get more out of Meeting. She offers suggestions for supporting teachers in Meeting as well. Protocols for two approaches students can use to center themselves in Meeting are shared by Chip Poston. Mary Sidwell describes creative alternatives to the traditional Meeting format that add new energy to her school's Meeting for Worship. Elementary school teachers wanting to include Meeting or a special time for centering in their classrooms are given helpful tips and observations by Christie Duncan-Tessmer. Richard Brady reflects on the hidden dimension of Meeting for Worship.

The Quaker practice of worship sharing, described by McHenry is a corporate practice in which a contemplative space is created for considering a query together. Janet Chance describes clearness committees, another corporate contemplative practice that can help a teacher (or a student) discern how to proceed with a question or challenge. Finally, Marcy Seitel describes how mindfulness is nurtured in the context of a Friends school community through Meeting for Worship, the assessment process, town meeting, and other school practices.

Meeting for Worship: Developing Reflective Practice in Friends Schools

Irene McHenry

John Fothergill, an eighteenth-century British Quaker educator, posited that a goal for Friends education is "to habituate children, from their early infancy, to silence and attention," and that this habit will form "the ground-work of a well-cultivated understanding." All Friends schools hold Meeting for Worship, a regular practice in developing the habit of silence, attention, and reflection. From the Quaker viewpoint, Meeting is a time period in which the school community gathers together in silence with intention to be in a reflective, receptive mode, open to the divine spark within each person. Viewed through the lens of mindfulness practice, Meeting is a regular opportunity to practice centering, focusing attention with an alert and relaxed mind, developing the skills for expanding awareness of all that is present in the mind, spirit, and the gathered community.

Even though Meeting for Worship is predominantly a group experience of collective silence, the Quaker aspect of Meeting includes inspirational speaking. When a person feels "led to speak," he or she stands and offers the message in a clear voice. The message may be in the form of a contemplative thought, an image, a song, a poem, a memory, an observation, a question. The group is expected to settle into a period of silent reflection before another message is offered. Occasionally, one person's message may prompt others to offer a message, and sometimes a theme emerges within the group. Meeting ends with each person in the group shaking hands with his or her neighbor.

Kim Hays' research on Quaker high schools shows that, from a student perspective, Meeting for Worship is a time for self-reflection and relational reflection. Unique to Quaker pedagogy is the cultivation of an ongoing habit of personal reflection and shared community reflections. Because Friends have neither doctrines nor dogma, they place most emphasis on the manner in which people lead their lives and treat one another. This aspect, as well as the sense of genuine inquiry, allows young people from all religious traditions (or none) to feel comfortable together during the silence of a Friends school Meeting for Worship. A chance to imagine, to dream, to wonder, to solve a problem, to relax, and to listen to one another's thoughts awaits members of a school community during Meeting for Worship. Meeting provides an opportunity for everyone to gain fresh perspectives on daily life.

In Friends schools, the school community (or division, or classroom) generally gathers weekly for school Meeting for Worship. Sitting still in silence can be difficult or uncomfortable for children and teenagers if there is no orientation to the practice. Teachers in Friends schools use many techniques to prepare their students for the experience of Meeting and spend time talking with them about ways to use the silence, how to center, how to listen. The goal is to cultivate an understanding that the silence is alive, that it is a time for settling and clarity, and that it helps to create a sense of community. Both the individual and the community grow within the silence as clarity is developed. Some simple strategies, as illustrated in the examples below, can support students in developing the core mindfulness skills for centering and reflection during Meeting for Worship. These skills are also key to learning. These strategies can be used in any classroom, whether or not in a Friends school, as activities to develop reflection, concentration, awareness, observation, and centered relaxation. The ideas came from educators at Friends Council workshops and in the Education Concerns Group of Philadelphia Yearly Meeting.

Very Young Children and Elementary School-Age Children

These practices are for short periods of silence each day that can support children in developing a tolerance for sitting still.

- Begin the day by having everyone hold hands and "pass a squeeze" while they all sit quietly. The length of time can be extended each day.

- Practice "building the silence" by having the class sit or stand in a circle in a darkened room. Pass a lit candle from one to another, carefully listening to the silence and focusing on the light while the candle makes it entirely around the circle.

- Use a jar of muddy water (with some glitter thrown in!) on a sunny windowsill. Shake the jar and suggest that our minds are like the jar of muddy water; we must let our busy, wild thoughts settle to let the Light shine through with clarity. Remind students that it takes time and practice. Alternatively, with children sitting in a circle, shake a jar of sand and water and place it in the center of the floor. Ask the students to settle themselves while the sand settles itself from the water.

- Give children a piece of colored string as they enter one of the first Meetings for the year. Suggest that each color denotes an idea, such as brown for the earth, white for peace. Encourage children to focus their thoughts on their string's color and share what comes to mind.

- For four-, five-, and six-year-olds, read *Daniel Goes to Meeting*, which describes Meeting for Worship and thoughts a small boy has and what he does during Meeting. Then try sitting in silence for a minute or two. After the main Meeting for Worship, students can write what they thought of and did during Meeting. Young children can dictate to teachers and then make an illustration. These sharings can become a class book.

- As a class group, on the way to Meeting for Worship do a walking meditation around school grounds (use a bell to stop every two to three minutes to observe). Stop and listen in silence to the natural sounds in the environment and observe the details of nature.

- For young children, present Meeting for Worship as a listening time. Have students imagine that they are out in the woods somewhere with animals such as deer and rabbits nearby. Ask them to get their bodies still enough so that the deer or rabbit would walk by not knowing that they were there. As they begin to get still, ask them to listen for sounds in the room. Then ask them to listen to the noises and the silence out-of-doors. Can they hear traffic? Wind? Finally, ask them to listen to their own breathing and notice how it is going in and out. Point out that once you get very still you can hear a lot of things you would not normally hear. Explain that in a silent meeting you might be able to hear messages within you that you would not normally hear.

- For second- and third-graders, stop all classroom activity 15 minutes before Meeting for Worship. Introduce the word *Listen* and then rearrange the letters to spell *Silent*. Next, read part of *The Other Way to Listen* by Byrd Baylor.

- For kindergartners, read aloud *Everybody Needs a Rock*. After the story, pass around a box of rocks and have each child select one to hold while they think about the rock and the story during Meeting for Worship. After Meeting, invite the children to share impressions. Various tactile objects can be used for handling and focusing, such as pieces of colored beeswax, yarn, telephone wire, tiny fabric squares, things with interesting textures.

- At the beginning of the school year, read *We're Going to Meeting for Worship* to the class. Then, visit the Meetinghouse and sit in the class' assigned spot to practice getting comfortable. Practice having Meeting, but for a brief period of time.

- Give each child a natural object, such as a leaf, a horse chestnut, corn kernel, bean, or twig. Invite the children into ten minutes of silence to study their object and be ready to describe and identify it when it is put in a pile with all the others. After ten minutes, ask children to put their objects together in the center of the circle. For the next step, the children try to identify their own item. Discuss how they knew it was theirs; could they have picked it out without the help of the silence?

Middle School and High School Students

- Invite each student in one class, such as eighth-graders in middle school or seniors in upper school, to memorize a poem. Open every Meeting for Worship for the year with one student reciting a poem.

- Invite sixth-grade students (middle school) or ninth-grade students (upper school) to take turns closing Meeting by initiating the end-of-Meeting handshake. This student can then invite others to share their "After Thoughts"—anything that the students had been thinking about during worship but had not wanted to share. This practice increases the number of voices heard and builds confidence for speaking during Meeting for Worship.

- Reflect upon Meeting for Worship after returning to the classroom. Teachers may ask if anyone had wanted to speak but was too afraid and ask him or her to share the message in class. Older students and adults can be invited to talk about how they have used Meeting and what it has meant to them in their lives.

- Invite the class to do reflective writing prior to Meeting for Worship, such as five minutes' free writing on "What do I bring to Meeting for Worship?" Follow by discussion.

- Talk about Meeting for Worship as a unique opportunity that is not afforded to many people: the chance to sit quietly and notice thoughts and feelings without having to be on the way somewhere or trying to accomplish anything is quite special. Encourage students to try to find moments outside of school to practice this kind of contemplation.

Faculty

Appropriate modeling by the adults is always important. Teachers can have important, simple messages to share, and one does not have to be a Quaker or a member of any religious group to speak during Meeting. Teachers are encouraged to use the time for silent reflection to resist the impulse to scan the group of students with an eye toward student behavior and resist the temptation to use Meeting as a platform for teaching. A teacher who has truly used Meeting for Worship well will come out refreshed.

For new teachers, Friends schools provide a brief in-service on the background and value of Meeting for Worship to Quakers and in a Friends school. Seasoned faculty members can give a description of a typical Meeting.

- At a faculty meeting, ask teachers to reflect on times when silence has been important to them and why, and ask them to share these experiences. Then, settle into a period of silent worship for about fifteen minutes and close with a handshake.

- Invite faculty to share with each other using these two queries for reflection: How do I make time for reflection in my classroom? How do I introduce silent meeting to students in my class?

Love, Admiration, Respect:
Meeting for Worship in the Classroom

Christie Duncan-Tessmer

What is Meeting for Worship in a Friends school? What is worship?
A dictionary defines worship as a verb that means to love, admire,
respect greatly. Worship in a Friends school provides the opportunity
for this kind of communion—an opportunity for the gathered school
or classroom community to sit together in a space of admiration and
respect, wonder and awe; an opportunity for refection, for mindful
awareness of self and other and the larger picture of others in the world.

Children in elementary grades and younger don't have the same
kind of definitional boundaries that adults frequently have between
time for work, time for play, and time to be connected with a sense of
wonder and awe. For them, work, play, and a sacred space or sense of
wonder are all the same thing and it doesn't have to be named—it's just
living. The boundary that children define is between engagement in
meaningful activity and boredom. And Meeting for Worship, when it is
seen as a time when one just has to sit still, be quiet, and count ceiling
tiles for twenty minutes, is boring! Introducing and participating in
worship in a way that is meaningful, not boring, can be quite simple.
This essay provides some thoughts and concrete tools that can be used
by elementary school teachers in preparing for worship with children in
the classroom.

Questions to Start

The place—physical, temporal, emotional—that a classroom makes for
Meeting for Worship can vary quite a bit. Teachers new to Quakerism
may shy away from it altogether. Others may include it as a matter of
daily scheduling with no further thought. Some teachers may labor over
it; some may feel they simply don't have the time or the permission to
include worship. Wherever one is coming from, it may be helpful to
consider some basic questions about classroom Meeting for Worship
and ideas for implementing it. If some of these ideas feel too church-y
or New Age-y for you, don't use those ideas. Find something that feels
comfortable to you.

What is classroom Meeting for Worship?

- It is time spent in the classroom centering down and reaching inward to that which unites each of us. It is time to focus on the wonder, joy, and love that fills the world and all that is in it.
- It is a moment of silence to refocus on what is important.
- It is time to appreciate the gifts and presence of each individual in the class.

Does it have to be silent and still?

- No! Sing! Make something! Dance, go for a walk, tell stories, play with clay, write a poem, play a game, draw, build!
- Parker Palmer writes, "One does not apply worship to life. You make it your practice until worship and life become one." This describes children and worship beautifully—it is exactly what young children already do.

Why should I squeeze one more thing into my crazy-busy day?

- Because your day is crazy and busy. And so is the kids' day. Is crazy-busy really what you want your classroom life to be about?
- Because you can focus more effectively in the midst of busyness if your mind and heart are settled.

When is a good time to have Meeting for Worship in the classroom?

- Every morning to start the day.
- Every Monday to start the week.
- When the class is struggling with something important or difficult.
- On a child's last day of school when they are transferring.
- To focus before a test, a performance, or an athletic event.
- When kids are overwrought.

Where?

- In your classroom.
- With another class in their room.
- In the Meetinghouse.
- In the library, auditorium, or gym.
- Outside in a field or a grotto or under a tree, in a garden or on a walking path.

- In a special classroom, such as art or music.
- Change your space once in a while. New settings are inspiring both for your planning ideas and for the kids' experience.

Set up?

Make the space special; mark the time as something out of the ordinary. You can do this just by adding a little something that you don't usually have in your room. Doing the same thing every time helps set this time apart as its own special event. For example:

- Ask the children to be silent as they enter the room.
- Light a candle.
- Sing a particular song to start or finish.
- Put some seasonal flowers in a special vase.
- Try some incense.
- Ring a bell, tap some wind chimes, or play an instrument to start.
- Take your shoes off.
- Sit on the floor if you are usually in chairs, or vice versa.

How long?

- 30 seconds; 5 minutes; 30 minutes. It depends more on the age of the children and the context of the worship than an outside standard. Traditional silent worship will likely be shorter than worship through stories, discussion, and art.
- You may want to have an expectation of how long silent worship will be from the outset. On the other hand it can be powerful to simply worship as long as you are led to. Feel for the right moment to end it—not by how long the wiggliest child can stand it but by what seems right in the center of your self.
- Allow one of the children to determine when to break worship by shaking the hand of her neighbor. Being the one to determine when is the right time to end worship makes one have to pay very close attention!

Inspiration for Planning?

If your goal is to make space to live out of the Spirit for the duration of worship, then the plans for the structure of that worship need to come from the same place. Use all the additional resources you like, but start by taking time to sit quietly, centering yourself. Use

your heart to listen for guidance about what to do to make a space
for connection, reverent communion, and inward reflection in your
classroom. Then, if you need to complement or support your leadings
with resources, turn to friends and co-workers; stories; books about
worship, centering, meditation; craft resources.

Introducing Centering to Children

Wherever you are led to go with your class in worship, whether you
lead a simple minute of traditional silent worship, include a story and
discussion, or create a whole community service endeavor rising out of
worship, the experience needs to start from a centered, spiritual space.
That traditional "moment of silence" needs to be a meaningful centering
into the wisdom and love that unites and feeds us.

You may have had the experience of walking into a worship service,
whether Quaker or not, and feeling deeply that there is something
electric or binding moving through the room. The worship pulls you
right into the center of it. However, a classroom (or a Meetinghouse) full
of children who are not experienced in worship in the manner of Friends
is not likely to start at such a powerful place. So we can provide a bit
of a map to guide ourselves and our children to be open to the Spirit.
Following are a few suggestions of landmarks for your map. Teaching
landmarks to the children and starting with the same routine every time
will help them learn how to use the time and eventually to sink naturally
into worship as soon as they start to gather.

The first several times you worship with a class (more for younger
children, less for older, but always more than once), be explicit, in
language meaningful to you, about what Meeting for Worship is about.
Keep it simple; for example:

- We're going to listen with our hearts.
- We're going to let go of everyday thoughts and concentrate on
  what is most important deep inside of us.
- We're going to be still and feel the love that is inside and all around
  each of us.

By not getting too specific, you allow the children to recognize love by
their own understanding. By using words you may not use all the time,
such as love, you set this time apart as something special.

Teach the children explicitly how to sit. Here's a way to explain appropriate posture during worship:

> The way we respectfully and reverently hold ourselves physically is significant. We do not sit all slouched over like we do when we're watching any old show on TV. We sit up, in a balanced way. When our bodies are balanced, it helps us find internal balance as well. Sitting with straight spines, relaxed and regal but not stiff like soldiers, allows our breath to be natural and deep.

I like to draw attention to hands. As soon as I start talking about sitting straight and centering down, children start holding their hands in traditional Buddhist meditation positions and then they start giggling. When I ask them what they think about when they do that the answers are frequently about cartoons. I explain that serious meditators hold their hands in different ways because hands are powerful and when they put their thumb and forefinger together it means something to them. To the kids, however, it just means cartoons. So I show them how I hold my hands in a way that is meaningful to me: open in my lap to remind me to be open to any gift of a thought or idea or feeling or song that may be waiting for me in worship. This also helps children to be aware of restless hands in worship and gives them something to do with them.

The older children are, the less they want to close their eyes. The benefit of closing one's eyes is that every movement and every friend in sight does not catch one's attention; rather, attention is drawn internally. An alternative is to look down at the floor a foot or so in front of oneself.

Centering into silence is made easier with a focus on breathing, a natural process. Suggest starting with a deep breath. It is amazing how relaxing and cleansing and centering such a simple thing can be.

Using the God Word with Kids

It is not unusual for teachers to hesitate to bring up issues of spirituality and divinity with students. Those who have had experience in public schools have learned that it is inappropriate to bring up such matters in the classroom. On the other hand, Friends schools have made a commitment to supporting the spiritual growth of children, typically both in their written statements and in their actions. For this reason, teachers are invited to explore ways to bring the spiritual into the classroom explicitly and implicitly.

- That which is Divine has many names. Use the ones that are comfortable to you:

    Love

    Spirit

    Force of Good

    Divine

    Light

    Creative spirit

    Nature

    Source

    Encourage the children to use the names comfortable to them.

- If you share your beliefs, do it very briefly. Your speaking *briefly* guards against their absorbing your beliefs as their own, without doing the spiritual work they need to do.

- If students are asking questions that feel too personal to you, don't hesitate to tell them that your faith is personal and you choose not to share more than you already have. Allow them the same option.

- Encourage them to speak with their family about what their family beliefs and traditions are. Make space for them to share with each other what their beliefs and traditions are.

- Some kids don't believe in Spirit. Their beliefs need to be welcomed as safely as every other religious belief the children bring into the classroom. This is one reason for using names for God that are less connected to religious traditions: Love, Wisdom, Truth (all names Quakers like to use!).

Living from the Center

In the beginning of this essay, I stated that children don't separate regular, everyday space from sacred space in their lives. Now I've written a whole essay about providing support for making one part of the day, worship, sacred. This is a segmented way of perceiving worship and it may be used in that way. Alternatively, however, worship can be understood as one more part of the life-filled day where particular care is given to recognizing that life. Next on the daily schedule may be math class, which is also part of the life-filled day where particular attention is given to numbers and their patterns. Regardless of the content of one's interactions (numbers, music, places and events, centering), the life that courses through and unites each of us in a fundamental, unseen way is present. The reaching and the searching are truly something that can be part of each breath we take.

On a very long car ride across several states when my daughter was four, she announced, "I'm God and you're God and that tree is God, we're all just different shapes." Less than a minute later, with just as much gravity, she announced, "Wouldn't it be funny if walkie-talkies were phones that walked?" In her perception, walkie-talkies, trees, her self and God are all of a piece. Math, language arts, and social studies are of that same piece. The way in which we approach these subjects and our friends who are learning about them is just as much a matter of making space for perceiving the Divine as is worship. Children already do this—in this way the children can be our teachers.

How Shall I Use My Time in Meeting for Worship?

Chip Poston

The protocol presented here has been used by student leaders at George School for orienting students in grades nine through twelve to the Quaker practice of Meeting for Worship, a weekly gathering of the whole school community. In using or adapting this protocol in your school, the student leaders should decide ahead of time who will read or explain the material to the group, which meditation you will use first, and who will lead it.

What Is Meeting for Worship?

Reader #1: The main purpose of these sessions is to help you understand what happens in a Quaker Meeting for Worship and to help you to use your time there meaningfully. Friends believe that each of us has an "inward teacher," or a "light within," which most of us experience as the voice of our conscience. Being still in order to listen to our "inward teacher" is the most important part of the Meeting for Worship.

Although our Meetings are based in silence, Friends believe that anyone who has a message to share may rise and speak in Meeting. We try to come to Meeting "with heart and mind prepared." Then we listen for the spirit of truth inside us. If we feel we are given a message to share with the group, we rise and speak. Sometimes no one will speak during an entire Meeting. The silence itself can be healing and nourishing.

Reader #2: For many people, sitting in silence may be difficult— especially in the beginning. It is difficult! In a Friends school, the Meeting for Worship comes in the middle of a busy day of classes and other obligations, where both teachers and students are working hard. During the school day we have many distractions, pressures and disappointments. It is only natural to bring our restlessness into the silence with us.

So at times being still in Meeting for Worship may seem like hard work. Quaker worship is like an art, and like every art it has its own technique and needs continual practice—trying, failing, and trying again—before we are successful. And as with any other art, the learning is never finished.

Reader #1: Many of us are uncomfortable with silence. We get bored and restless, and we don't know what to do with our time in Meeting. Our restlessness may in turn disturb others. If we end up simply watching the clock in Meeting, the time can pass very slowly indeed!

At this time, leaders can share with the group how they use their time in Meeting, then ask experienced members of the group to speak to the same question.

Making the Transition into Silence

Reader #2: The following technique has helped others to be still in Meeting. We want to practice it together for a few minutes in the form of a meditation.

Meditation A: The Sacred Word

Begin by choosing a "sacred word" to help you reflect deeply and quietly during Meeting. The sacred word can be a part of your religious tradition or just a word that you feel comfortable with. Examples include Lord, One, Allah, Peace, Love, Shalom, Jesus, Truth, Buddha. Having chosen a sacred word, stick with it during our practice session— although you may change to a different sacred word or phrase later on.

Settle into a comfortable position with your back straight, both your feet flat on the floor, and your eyes closed. (If you are uncomfortable with closing your eyes, you can open them slightly and fix them on a point on the floor a few feet in front of you.) Then begin to repeat your sacred word to yourself silently; use it to help you reflect deeply and quietly during Meeting.

If you become aware of distracting thoughts, gently return to your sacred word. Remember that thoughts are normal during meditation; you are not trying to prevent them. But thoughts can be like boats floating down a river. We can be aware of their passing, but if we find ourselves getting carried away by certain thoughts, we gently remind ourselves to return to the sacred word.

Now: Let's practice this technique together for the next two minutes. *(After two minutes, slowly end and give a chance for feedback.)*

Meditation B: Breath Awareness

Reader #1: The following technique has helped others to be still in Meeting. We want to practice it together for a few minutes in the form of a guided meditation.

Get into a comfortable position with your back straight and your eyes closed.

Now, become aware of the sensation of your breathing as the air passes through your nostrils. Feel its touch. Notice where in your nostrils you feel the touch of the air when you inhale *(pause)* and when you exhale *(pause)*.

Do not try to control your breathing. This is not an exercise in breathing but in awareness. So if your breathing is shallow, leave it that way. Do not interfere with it. Just observe it.

If it is helpful, you can count your breaths. See if you can maintain your awareness of breathing from your first to your tenth breath. Many people cannot! If you reach ten, begin with one again and keep counting. You might count to yourself, "In one, out one...in two, out two."

Try to maintain the awareness of each breath you take for the next several minutes. If you are distracted, gently return to your breathing as soon as you become aware of your wandering.

(After two minutes, slowly end the exercise and see if there is any feedback from the group.)

Reader #2: At first, you may spend most of your time in Meeting learning how to settle down, or "center down" as some Friends say. Regardless of how you try to settle down you may find it difficult. Remember what we said earlier about practicing the "art" of Meeting for Worship. It is somewhat like learning to play a sport or developing math skills. You should expect it to be difficult in the beginning, but it will grow easier as you practice. Some weeks it will be easier than others. The most important thing is that you make a sincere effort each time you are in Meeting.

Are there any questions?

Helpful Pointers for Meeting for Worship

At this point the leaders can invite the group to brainstorm what makes for a good Meeting for Worship. See if they can come up with everything on the following list. (If not, you can read them and ask the group how each contributes to a more valuable Meeting for Worship.) As the group brainstorms, be sure to explain the reasons for each, as the reasons aren't often evident to those new to Meeting for Worship. Please do your best to address each of the points listed below.

1. Come into Meeting quietly. The Meeting for Worship begins as soon as the first person enters the Meetinghouse, and often the quality of a Meeting is related to how quietly it begins. Please do not disturb others as they worship. If you must leave before Meeting is over, go quietly.

2. Sit appropriately. Find a comfortable position with your back straight. Many Friends also find it helpful to close their eyes during Meeting. These two simple acts can help you to become calm in body, mind, and spirit. Please do not put your feet on the benches, just as you wouldn't in a church, synagogue, or mosque. The Meetinghouse is a place of worship.

3. Listen deeply. Meeting is a quiet time for listening to the "inward teacher." Please do not whisper or talk with friends during Meeting and do not read during Meeting. Avoid any behavior that might disturb others.

4. Come to Meeting "with heart and mind prepared." Friends do not go to Meeting with a prepared speech; nor do we go determined either to speak or not to speak. We speak when we are moved by the Spirit within. However, you can bring to Meeting other people's ideas that you have found meaningful. These ideas may help others. Words from the Bible and from Quaker history are often used in this way by Friends. It's fine—and appropriate—to share significant thoughts, ideas, or stories from your own experience and study.

5. Work to "tune in," to the "feel" of the Meeting, which is deeper than your individual thoughts. If you give too much attention to your own ideas and emotions you may not be able to realize the shared experience of the Meeting for Worship.

6. Be open to speaking in Meeting! Messages in Meeting are usually brief statements of insight, inspiration, or concern. Often when people feel called to speak in Meeting, they feel their heart begin to beat rapidly. If you feel called to speak, speak! Speak loudly enough so that you may be heard by everyone in the Meetinghouse—it's a large room!

7. Allow for a time of reflection between messages. Every message should be followed by a time of at least several minutes of silence. Meeting for Worship is a time for listening, not for discussion or debate. Remember that you can learn from messages with which you may not agree.

8. Shake hands with others at the end of Meeting. It's a good chance to greet friends and maybe make new ones.

9. Share your reactions with people who spoke in Meeting. If you appreciated someone's message, tell her or him so. The feedback will mean a lot.

End with a moment of silence together; then shake hands.

Adapted from the curriculum Orientation to Quakerism and Meeting for Worship *by Chip Poston, available for download from www.friendscouncil.org.*

Opening a World of Silence

Mary B. Minor Sidwell

The traditions of beginning and ending our days at Olney Friends School with ten minutes of silence and of having twice-weekly Meetings for Worship are of enduring importance. Olney Friends School is a small, boarding high school in the hills of southeastern Ohio founded by Quakers in 1837. On the face of it, one might imagine Olney to be rural and lacking in diversity. Half of that is true. The school is situated on 350 acres of farmland and forest. What often surprises visitors is that the student body is about 40 percent international; 12 countries are represented in the 2008 school community. One of the challenges is helping students and new staff to become open to the rich world of silent meditation. For a diverse school community, with representatives of many cultures and countries, quiet meditation often becomes meaningful on many levels.

Several times during the year volunteers who serve on the Spiritual Life Committee suggest a more guided use of the longer, forty-minute silent meetings. This committee, composed of both adults and students, is often creatively inspired as they strive to help the community find useful practice and meaning in the quiet times. What follows are a few of the activities used during the school year.

- In one exercise, small pieces of paper and a pencil are placed on the circle of chairs, instructions communicated (often by a student), and then time allowed for thoughts to be quietly expressed. We are asked to look two seats to the left and write down something we appreciate about that person (assuring everyone receives a note). Then notes may be written to others in the room, particularly to those with whom we may not have verbally communicated often. These "appreciations" are handed to the subject after Meeting ends.

- Before Thanksgiving we often place a colorful blanket in the middle of the floor. Ahead of time, we ask those who wish to bring an object that represents something for which they are thankful to place on the blanket. If one feels moved to speak out of the silence, such communications are encouraged.

- Recently, long rolls of paper and colored markers became canvas for artistic expressions about the subject of "community." Blank outlines of a mandala may be offered and then each quietly filled with colors, allowing for a break from the focus of the academic day.

- A meeting for singing is often a welcome change before Christmas vacation begins or during the cold days of winter.

Several weeks into the school year, the Spiritual Life Committee was curious about how students were making use of the silence during Meeting for Worship. Again, small pieces of paper and pencils were distributed. Those present at mid-week Meeting were asked to write briefly on that subject, their thoughts to remain anonymous. A few samples follow:

All problems dissolve in love, so I try to use the silence to dissolve in love.

The silence gives me time to pray for others, for myself, for the world, for situations, for couples, for love, for relationships....time to reflect on what is good, where I need help, what I could do differently, how I can help, memories, good & bad....time to collect my thoughts, my feelings, my to-do list.

I will sometimes pray for each person in the room, or find qualities I like about them, and my favorite so far, is to look around the room at each person and think about how they have humbled me or what I have learned from them since I have been here. Sometimes when I pray for myself I will ask for better relationships with certain people or the strength to do something hard. And lately I have needed help prioritizing and help with school and getting the energy to do everything I need to do. And I know God will help. It comes in funny ways sometimes, but he comes.

The silence gives me space and time that forces reflection. It drains away emotion, allowing me to see things more clearly.

Only what is real can exist in the silence. You can see truth in a communal way in the silence that you cannot see otherwise. Silence unwinds the lies we tell ourselves and each other. It sets us free.

Thus out of these regular, quiet times of reflection in our school community come insight and clarity, along with unique learning that is so valuable in a world where silence is unusual.

The Magic Eye:
Tuning In During Meeting for Worship

Richard Brady

I'm sitting in Meeting for Worship and thinking back to an experience of two hours earlier.

I arrive in the Math Office and find an email waiting for me. It has the URL of the Chaco Canyon "Magic Eye" picture he mentioned to me the day before (http://www.eyetricks.com/3dstereo50.htm). At first sight it's just a wall of red, grey, and brown stones. I know there's something hidden here but I have trouble seeing any sign of it. The reflection of the overhead light on the monitor screen distracts me. I turn out the lights and sit gazing with eyes unfocused until I finally begin to see a small, three-dimensional patch. Holding onto that piece of the image, I try to let the surrounding area come into alignment. One feature remains indistinct. Moving away from the image, I see the last section come into sharp focus and I sigh in amazement.

I had no idea what I was looking for in the Magic Eye pictures, but I found it. In fact, when I think about the most important things I've found in my life—my life partner, my spiritual path, Sidwell Friends School—in none of these cases did I know what I was looking for.

Meeting for Worship is like that. When I arrive, I seldom know what I'm looking for. I'm often as surprised by the insights that arise within me as those coming from hearing the messages of others. Occasionally, I arrive at Meeting with a problem I want to think through. It may occupy my mind for all or most of the silent meeting, and I may find a resolution. But seldom is this a true insight. Insights are more likely to show up when I'm able to stop thinking up a solution and simply sit mindfully with my problem, "hold it in the Light" as Friends say. This process is a lot like seeing the third dimension in a Magic Eye picture. I can't figure it out. Someone else can't show it to me. I need to be patient and let it arrive.

In my classroom I post a Magic Eye Picture of the Week. When I get to class, a group of students is invariably clustered around it. Some have looked at similar pictures for years and have never seen a hidden image, yet they keep coming back to look at new ones. Are they drawn by the challenge and mystery of it?

I reflect on the challenge and mystery of finding something of value in Meeting for Worship. I've often heard students say they find more in Meeting as they grow older. I wonder about this. Do they become more patient? Make more of an effort to eliminate distracting reflections on their Meeting monitors by quieting and centering themselves? Perhaps they become more attentive to things they weren't looking for. Or maybe it's simply that Meeting has become a refuge for them, a place to de-stress, to stop all the thinking we do in our fast-paced Quaker upper school and truly rest. Occasionally, I have that experience. At the end of Meeting it feels as though my mind has been given a most refreshing bath.

This is what I yearn for in Meeting. Though I'm moved by many of the messages I hear there, it's the silence that provides me the opportunity to take these messages or my own ruminations to a place of inner stillness, to dwell with them and let other dimensions have a chance to reveal themselves. That is the real magic of Meeting for Worship.

Worship Sharing: Centering and Reflective Inquiry in Friends Schools

Irene McHenry

Worship sharing is a reflective practice that calls for clear focus on a specific topic or query. In the context of developing mindfulness skills, worship sharing provides experiential practice in centering into silence, focusing on one guiding thought or image, and re-centering into silence after each person's spoken message. In the context of Quaker practice, worship sharing is similar to Meeting for Worship in that each spoken message is a gift wrapped in silent reflection. The difference between speaking in Meeting for Worship and speaking during worship sharing is that in worship sharing each person takes a turn to speak and there is one common focus for the gathering.

Use of the query is a traditional Quaker practice for in-depth contemplation and examination of how we are living our lives, individually and in community. Quakers value knowing experientially. The query, a Quaker tool for reflection, lends itself perfectly to an educational setting. A query is a special kind of question with no quick, easy, or obvious yes or no answer. Friends use queries to explore an issue and share the depth of their understanding with each other. In a school setting, queries used in classes and faculty meetings inspire reflection while building an atmosphere of respectful listening and dialogue. To create a query that is accessible to children at various developmental stages, it is essential to begin by talking with students about the concept of a query and providing some examples. Students of all ages can develop their own queries for use in classroom Meeting and worship sharing in small groups. Below are some examples of queries developed for students of various ages.

Queries for Young Children:

- How can I remain peaceful if people around me are fighting?
- How many toys are enough? Do I have enough or too many or too few?

Queries for Middle School Students:

- How can I resolve conflict in my own life and how does this knowledge inform the resolution of conflict in the world?
- How can I help to keep the environment healthy and beautiful for myself and others?

Queries for High School Students:

- How do I keep my own integrity while being open in dialogue to the difference that might change my point of view?
- Is war the greatest evil human beings commit against each other?

Students of any age are quite adept at formulating their own queries. In some Friends schools, each class takes a turn formulating a query for a larger group cither for worship sharing or for Meeting for Worship. Some Friends schools have committees of students and faculty at each division level to look after the spiritual life of the school. These committees are a good source for developing queries. An excellent source for queries is the Faith and Practice document from any Yearly Meeting of the Religious Society of Friends (many of these documents can be found on the web). Another valuable resource is the Friends Council's publication *Advices and Queries for Friends School Community Life*.

A Protocol for Introducing Worship Sharing

Worship sharing begins with silent centering. It works well if everyone is seated in a circle. The teacher is a participant in the circle. The teacher (for younger children) or the leader (good leadership opportunity for middle-school and upper-school students) briefly describes worship sharing practice. Following are the main points:

- Worship sharing is focused around a topic or query (a special question for reflection with no obvious yes or no answer).

- The leader reads the focus topic or query out loud to the group after the opening silent worship time and asks at least one other person to read it aloud as well, so that the gathered group has the opportunity to hear it read by more than one voice. The query could also be printed on small cards for each person to hold.

- Each person has a turn to share. A person may "pass," if that feels right. Everyone takes a turn to share before anyone shares a second time. (It can be useful to pass a beautiful object, such as a seashell or a Native American "talking stick," so that it is clear when the object reaches you, it is your turn to speak. Another idea is to use an object related to the query, for example, a paper crane for peace, a leaf or flower for stewardship.)

- When one person is speaking, everyone directs all of his or her attention to listening to the words of the speaker with open mind and heart. This is not a time for discussion, reaction, or debate. Each person's sharing is an offering to be received without judgment. Responses may be shaped in part by previous speakers; however, all responses should be directly to the query, not to what others have said. The most meaningful response to each sharing is respectful, silent reflection.

- Worship sharing ends by returning to a period of silent reflection. The end of the reflection is marked by the shaking of hands, just as in the end of Meeting for Worship.

Mindful Discernment:
The Clearness Process

Janet Chance

When you see the word *mindfulness*, what do you imagine? Some may hear the gentle toning of a bell, rippling outward, as individuals pause in their slow, circuitous path around a bamboo grove; some may visualize a woman, centering on her breath as she exhales; some might follow a flicker of incense to a space of calm.

In this essay, I describe another, perhaps less familiar practice to add to this repertoire of imaginings: the clearness process. *Clearness* is a special focus-group process for individual discernment conducted in the spirit of Quaker inquiry. The clearness committee process became a part of spiritual practice in the 1660s, a mere decade after the Society of Friends (or Quakers) originally emerged. Clearness process continues to be a vibrant aspect of Quakerism, at both the local (or Monthly Meeting) level and the national (Yearly Meeting) level, and is most commonly used on two occasions: when couples consider entering into a life partnership and when individuals apply for membership within the Society of Friends. In recent years, clearness process gained appreciation outside of Quaker circles when visionaries such as Parker Palmer introduced it to public educators through his Courage to Teach program.

Clearness process is a simple, elegant practice, that invites a "focus person" to welcome and attend to his or her inner teacher (or inner light, as Quakers often say) within the support and care of a small group of attentive listeners, usually four to six people. One of the most important understandings is the agreement to maintain double confidentiality: everything that takes place in the committee will remain confidential, and no one will discuss the issue with the focus person afterward, unless invited to do so by the focus person. The group is encouraged to welcome meditative silence throughout the process: the focus person speaks out of silence, the process ends with silence, and the group is encouraged to allow for generous periods of silence throughout. After selecting a facilitator to guide the process and a note-taker to record only the questions for later reflection, the group settles into silence. When moved to do so, the focus person begins by briefly describing his or her question or concern, including any background or detail that may be necessary so that listeners can understand the question. In my experience, these questions are usually about work or relationships or some combination of the two. Here are two examples of the kind of issues or concerns that might be raised:

- *I've just learned that my sister has terminal cancer. How do I support her right now, while still keeping up with everything else?*

- *One of my students is struggling because his parents are in the midst of a divorce. He is having difficulty in geometry, and I think he might have a learning difference, but his parents are reluctant to have him tested and don't seem to have much time for him right now. I'm at my wit's end.*

After listening and asking any brief factual questions, the group proceeds to ask open-ended questions to the focus person, with the emphasis on holding the person's concern aloft in order to provide support so she can hear his or her inner teacher. The group takes care neither to offer advice nor to ask questions that are actually advice in disguise. Instead, the group asks questions that support the focus person in attending to his or her own inner wisdom, and so the open-ended questions that emerge may be unconventional, indirect, or even somewhat surprising.

- *The last time you spoke with your sister, what topics came up?*

- *What are this student's unique interests or talents?*

Toward the end of the clearness process, the focus person chooses whether or not to request that others "mirror" in addition to asking deepening questions. Mirroring often involves reflecting back body language or gestures that the focus person used, such as the following:

- *Your words were louder and more rushed whenever you mentioned your sister's oldest child.*

- *I noticed that you grinned whenever you mentioned your student's penchant for puns and riddles.*

Finally, the committee ends the clearness process with celebrations, affirming the group's work together, with comments such as these:

- *Thanks for asking me that question about the last time I spoke with my sister; it reminded me of something I had forgotten.*

- *I felt moved by how well you know this student.*

Like other forms of mindfulness, the clearness committee process is counter-cultural in several respects. In our culture, we tend to "consume" space, and interruption can be a common, even expected, part of conversational discourse. In many educational settings, for example, students leap into discussions quickly, often before they have had time to reflect, a habit that is encouraged by the pace of dialogue. It is almost as if contributing to discussions is more important than the quality or thought that is present within the contribution. Similarly, "winning" the argument is often given more value than listening to various insightful perspectives. In contrast, clearness process invites participants to become comfortable with silence amid and between the asking of questions. Acquiring comfort with the silence in clearness process can be challenging, even for those familiar with Meeting for Worship, perhaps because we habitually and unknowingly connect the act of asking questions to filling space.

A related aspect of clearness process, common to every mindfulness practice, is that participants are asked to approach it from a nonjudgmental stance. As with allowing silence, this approach involves a kind of retraining and newfound awareness. In my experience, logical and analytical questions rarely seem open enough in the clearness context; questions feel more meaningful if I allow them to "bubble up" from a place of integrated awareness, combining all aspects of the self: heart, body, mind, and spirit. One of the profound features of developing this kind of listening awareness, which feminist writers have referred to as "listening with," is that it both draws upon and strengthens a person's sense of empathy. In clearness practice, we learn how to care more deeply: for our true selves, by listening to our inner teacher apart from other distractions, and for others, by listening attentively and honoring another's spirit. As such, this practice fits quite comfortably within a relational approach to ethics, as envisioned by Nel Noddings in *The Challenge to Care in Schools.*

Clearness process, then, is a reflective practice, a journey. Like all such practices, it is about much more than it initially seems. While the focus person shares a deeply held concern, there is not actually an extrinsic goal, such as fixing a problem; instead, there is an open-ended sense that no one knows what will emerge, that a completely new set of questions may emerge from the original question.

Prior to holding a clearness committee, it is helpful to review the process with participants, even when they have experienced it before, because of the shift in awareness that clearness process requires. As a member of a clearness committee, the one way I've found to "step in" gently is to request that the group pause for some silent reflection. This creates a space for everyone to center, regardless of whether the issue is that the pace of questions is too rushed or the questions are veering into advice. Furthermore, anyone in the group, including the focus person, can easily make a request for silent reflection without causing disruption to the group's sense of trust. Afterward, creating space for group reflection on the process invites learning that connects to growth over time. Finally, and significantly, clearness process is an invitational experience; no one is ever required to be a focus person.

In reflecting on the clearness committee experience, many express the following:

- *Feeling honored to have been trusted with a matter of importance*
- *Closer connection to other members of the group*
- *Awareness that asking open-ended questions is challenging or unfamiliar*
- *Surprise at the power of such a simple process*
- *Recognition that they gained new insights*
- *Appreciation for the wisdom of each person's inner teacher*
- *Appreciation for the power of attentive listening*

Clearness process is currently used in a handful of Friends schools and Friends Council on Education programs. At Guilford College and in Westtown's upper school, clearness process provides the opportunity for students to reflect on one's life path: for example, in deciding which career to pursue after college. At The Meeting School in New Hampshire, clearness is a regular part of campus life; it is used for personal discernment, in the traditional manner of Friends, and a related practice, a hybrid of clearness and mediation, provides the opportunity for guided reflection when someone breaks a community agreement. Clearness is also an integral part of Friends Council on Education's SPARC (Spirited Practice and Renewed Courage) Program for educators. As more educators and young people experience the clearness process, it is exciting to imagine how this may ripple outwards, creating a new way of experiencing dialogue each day: not rushed or crowded, but energized, open, and vitally connected to the search for deeper understanding.

Mindfulness in a School Community

Marcy Baker Seitel

We often joke in middle school, "Oh, it's not all about me?" A focus on self is one of the hallmarks of early adolescence. Who am I? Do people like me? What is so special about me? Do I have anything to contribute to this life I'm part of? What does it all matter, anyway? In my work as teacher and administrator, I see these good existential questions as wonderful opportunities to foster mindfulness of self, a mindfulness that includes a full definition of a self that identifies with and contributes to a community. For an adolescent, being mindful of oneself as a community member becomes part of knowing oneself. The community must be a healthy, vibrant place if it is to have the role of eliciting good and true ideas and actions from its members. At Thornton Friends School's middle school, we have developed practices that foster both a rich community life and an authentic way for students to explore their own identities. Exploring self and community happen together through mindfulness practices.

At Thornton, shaping social life and shaping an individual go hand in hand. The community is not just the sum of individuals, but the place where individualities are recognized and realized. A student is never just an individual at school, even when we think in terms of teaching and assessing individual students. The student always exists in the interactive context of the school community. The qualities of individual and community are absolutely interdependent.

Envisioning, shaping, and tending this daily social forum is the work, the concern, and the joy of educators. Quakers are historically very ambitious when it comes to social relationships, and Quaker schools reflect this ambition. We believe it is possible to live peacefully in the world and seek peace wherever we go. A powerful way to make headway with this goal is to form a school community that is based on peace, respect, and care for one another, honoring individuality, practicing the interpersonal skills that bring satisfying resolutions to conflict, and together seeking inner guidance. It is in this community that we practice our hope of "finding that of God in one another."

At the heart of the shaping of individual selves and a community of young people who feel free to be themselves are practices that invite and foster mindfulness. At Thornton Friends School's middle school, we have practices that invite, encourage, and compel students to be mindful of their lives as community members. We ask our students to be mindful of many things at the same time—to be mindful of their inner thoughts and feelings, to feel compassion for their classmates, to understand the needs that a healthy community has, and to be aware that what we do at school is connected to the bigger community outside our school and to the world as a social place and a planet. If we do our work well, students will realize who they are and what they bring to the world and will live peacefully with one another at school. This knowledge of community life and the inner practices of community mindfulness, we hope, will bring real peace into our world.

Mindful Action

Mindfulness of the community can be seen in the way that students act in the school community. When students are not mindful of others, their behavior may be hurtful to the community. These behaviors include the following:

- Hurtful language, blaming, gossiping
- Impulsive reactions in word or deed
- Arguing without seeking resolution
- Promoting oneself without thought of the impact on others

Not all of these behaviors will necessarily get a student into "trouble" with the school, but all of them will lessen the quality of community life and make school a place where students will not feel safe to try new ideas and act as their authentic selves. Without safety and authenticity, the community suffers. On the other hand, behaviors that show mindfulness of the community strengthen community life; these behaviors include the following:

- Calm response to others, speaking using a clear, steady voice
- Self-control of behavior
- Accepting the intended and unintended consequences of one's own actions
- Questioning authority respectfully
- Stating views with the purpose of building understanding and finding solutions

- Turning to teachers, administrators, and parents for help, and offering help to others
- Using truthful and compassionate language, listening and acting empathically

Each of these behaviors contributes to the community being a safe and vibrant place. The heart of our program is to help students find their answers within themselves by getting to know themselves better. We guide students in creating a viable, safe, nurturing community so that everyone else can get to know themselves and each other. The building of community and the fostering of individual growth develop intertwined in one continuous process.

Mindfulness of the Self in Community

At our middle school, we devote ample time both to assessing our students and to asking our students to assess themselves. We see both kinds of assessments as central to helping middle schoolers become aware of who they are, how they are changing, and how they affect others. The school schedule reflects the importance of these assessments—six full days are set aside each year for this work.

We don't give grades. This frees us to assess the students in all of their many facets without ever having to average all of these facets into a letter grade. All aspects of student performance show growth or lack of growth, and that is what teachers write about in their progress reports. These reports are one- or two-paragraph narratives that students' families read carefully. Many big and small things are noted, and changes are asked for clearly.

Our assessments are designed and used to help the student grow as a "whole child," a person in the world with his or her own path and integrity. Along with the academic report come the advisor's comments, which give the student feedback on how he or she is growing as a person within the school community. Participating in class discussions, feeling safe to try new ideas, feeling focused and not distracted by the antics of others, accepting feedback as good and useful information instead of harsh criticism to be defended against—all of these phenomena are social and academic, and even more, they are very much part of preparing a young person to live in a very complicated world in a self-aware, caring, intentional way.

Advisors draw from comments made by other teachers and from direct observations of the student in all aspects of school life to write several paragraphs about each student. They comment on the student in the life of the school and the life with others. The purpose of the advisor's comments is to reflect back to a student the growth that the advisor has seen over the quarter in academic classes, at lunch, on fieldtrips, and in all aspects of the school life. They highlight strengths—enumerate and celebrate them—and ask for change in one or two areas of work or behavior. We hope that, with authentic reflections of themselves from a trusted adult they know well, students will more fully understand themselves and how they affect others and the life of the community. And with the reflection, the student becomes responsible to the community either to use a gift or to strengthen an area of weakness.

Twice a year students undertake a process of assessing their own work. Student self-assessment takes a period of several days at the end of each semester. Students first write a self-assessment, then create a portfolio of the work they deem to be their best for the semester. Finally, during a special conference, they present their written self-assessment to their parents or other loving adults in their lives and to their advisors. Even though the adults have read part or all of the self-assessment as it was written, it is different to sit together in a conference and hear the whole piece at one time.

We see the self-assessment process as the heart of our program for middle schoolers, and it is the most concrete practice we have for building mindfulness about academic work, personal growth, and growth in the school community. The amount of time devoted to this process tells teachers, students, and families that the process is a central part of the school's program. Just as their teachers and advisors do for the progress report, students assess their growth in each aspect of their program. They look at their growth in their five academic classes, physical education, the arts, fieldtrips, Meeting for Worship, community service, and community life, including jobs, advisories, and all the in-between times in a school day. They might notice that they are patient and friendly in one aspect of school but critical and irritable in another, or they might find one aspect of academics or community life very enjoyable and meaningful and another dimension pointless or not worth the effort asked. All of this is written about in detail.

Self-assessment begins with a series of questionnaires that students are asked to complete. The questions are sometimes quantitative, but most are reflective and give students the chance to examine their experience in each aspect of school life systematically. Students work on these assessments in each of their classes and in whole-school gatherings. The first questions are about the activities that the group experienced during the semester—the assignments, class activities, fieldtrips. Then they are asked to list the most memorable moments of the class. With these first two questions, students stand in the span of time of the whole semester, with the chance to see that their lives have been a journey through the semester.

The questions invite open reflection, such as: What did you learn that is important to you? What did you find to be most enjoyable about this class? What was especially challenging? How did you contribute to the learning of the class? Did you meet the behavior expectations of this class? Students are asked to think of examples to explain and clarify their more general answers. They are asked to be honest and specifically descriptive.

This is initially an uncomfortable process for new students. The teacher plays a role as friend and coach, and teachers and advisors reflect back to the student things they have seen and feel are important. These suggestions are only used if they feel true to the student.

After the different aspects of school life have all been examined, students are asked to write a couple of paragraphs about their overall experience. The conversations that advisors have with their students through this process are some of the best we have all year. Students have the time and space to think through their joys and frustrations with themselves and their community with the guide of an adult who cares about them deeply and can ask good guiding questions. Parents and other loving adults help their child at home, and in many cases, the conversations that come from this process give adults insights into their child's true experience in school above the day-to-day tasks and worries, to the overall experience of their own learning and development.

With the questions answered, the writing process goes back between student and advisor until it is complete and well written. The final product is a document that is a keepsake for the student and his or her family.

This process becomes easier for students with each semester. They know the questions and keep them in mind as they go through the semester. They come to talk about their experience day-to-day in the language of the self-assessment questionnaires—this is hard for me, this is challenging, or I think I'm doing really well in this area. These are statements of fact, not complaints or points of bragging. The self-assessment process gives students the vocabulary to describe their accomplishments, their discouragements, and the help they need to reach their goals. This is mindful academic and social life at its best. With the development of this vocabulary for inner experience, students can move into more mindful behaviors in community life. Because the whole school does the self-assessment process at one time, everyone is aware that self-assessment is a community process. As students feel their individuality, they look out at classmates and know that they, too, have strengths and challenges.

Corporate Practices to Support Community Life

The most important corporate practice is Meeting for Worship, which for our community takes place twice a week. Before we get to Meeting for Worship, our community gathers for attendance and announcements. It is very centering to hear the name of each student read off and to hear the quick but not always predictable replies of the students. The schedule for the day and the week are then reviewed—everyone in the community is thereby responsible for helping the schedule to work. Finally, teachers and students make announcements. Birthday wishes are sung, and accomplishments and good events are noted. If someone has a concern, he or she and their concern are "held in the light." Then we are ready for Meeting for Worship. We gather in silence, mindful of what the school week asks of us and mindful of the joys and worries that have been shared. We know that our life is rich, that we are not all alike in how we feel and what we are experiencing.

At the end of each day, students do jobs, such as vacuuming, organizing materials, and readying classrooms for the next day, and then come to "shake out." During this time, assignments are clarified and written in assignment books, announcements about the quality of clean up and things needed for the following day are made. When we are finished, students briefly show their assignment books to their advisors and then shake hands with the advisor. That is the end of the school day. We leave from our community gathering with students having organized themselves individually and collectively and with a final salutation to the advisor. Having the practice of gathering regularly to share information and make decisions that are appropriate for the students to make gives us an easy way to check in with students and know how they are doing with all of life's changes.

We have another forum for handling community life when things go wrong—our town meeting. These are held when there has been a hurtful action in the community. These things rarely happen, fortunately, but they are treated with care. A town meeting follows the process of worship sharing among Quakers. Participants are asked to share their experience and their thoughts, and not to respond to others' contributions. In a town meeting, not everyone is required to participate, but everyone is expected to. Through this process, students see how people are affected by a situation and how differently their schoolmates respond to the same situation. We simply hold each other in the Light.

Our community life is governed each day by a set of commitments.
- Fully participate in all class and school activities.
- Be prepared to do your best.
- Ask for help.
- Respect personal bubbles.
- Take ownership of yourself and your choices.
- Act and speak in a safe and kind way to yourself and others.

We hope that students will see these as the rules above our other more day-to-day rules. Taken together, our commitments give us a way of living our community life proactively to support everyone's participation and the common good.

Mindfulness in Community

I am here now,
In my body,
In my thoughts,
In my school community,
In my local community,
In the world.

One of the first steps in building mindfulness is building knowledge and awareness.

Our practices of assessment and self-assessment and of school Meetings and town meetings all help students focus on their own experience. At the same time, the different aspects of community life become illuminated—class discussions, class assignments, fieldtrips, lunchtime together. Once we have a vocabulary for talking about self-growth and about our community, we can all begin to learn from one another and to support one another. In a very real way, we all teach each other in community how to act in community. We reveal different possibilities and demonstrate outcomes to different kinds of actions or behavior.

When students leave our community, they take their knowledge of community life so that when they get into a social group, they will know that their own self-awareness is the starting point for learning about a new community. They will understand what they need to be successful, what they are comfortable with and what they are not comfortable with. Rather than reacting, they have within them the practice of being reflective and making decisions based on self-knowledge. We hope that their experiential knowledge about community will stay with them— that there is a structure to be looked for and understood. When students leave our middle school community, they feel they have a blueprint for navigating the more complicated community structures in high school. We send them off to find good in themselves, in their new campus or school, in their community, and in the world, and so to be active agents in making the world a better place for all of us.

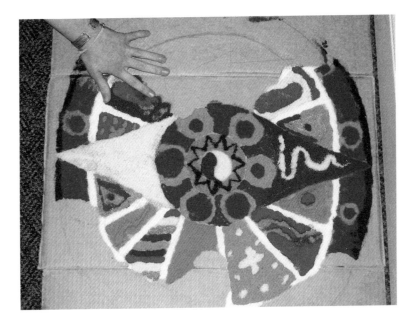

PART III
Cultivating Mindful Learning

Mindful learning refers to the development of a meta-awareness of the learning process while engaging in learning in any subject area. Mindful learning creates a context in which students can develop new insights, even wisdom. In this section teachers describe many ways in which they create mindful learning environments. One approach is to provide students with a time for stillness to help them center in order to be more fully present. This technique was described by Scattergood, McHenry, and Belasco in Part I and here by Becky Martin-Scull as she starts her classes with guided silence initiated by the use of a bell. Denise Aldridge also employs silence to help her students connect more deeply with nature through observation and drawing. Eric Mayer uses "noble silence" to help his students become more aware of all the present moment holds as they work together creating sand mandalas.

Mindfulness is used in a variety of forms to facilitate self-understanding. Questions or queries help students examine the role of grades in their learning process in Doug Tsoi's social studies classes. Hope Blosser uses questions to invite students in her English classes to look inward and then write about their lives. Martin-Scull employs guided visualizations to help her students develop a healthy relationship to negative emotions. She also invites students to take a personal question into silence, holding it "in their hearts" and waiting for an answer to emerge. Richard Brady uses *lectio divina*, or holy reading and journal writing, to help his students deepen their connection to poems and prose passages. Self-understanding is also facilitated by the listening that students give to and receive from their peers. The experience of being listened to and listening without judgment enables those sharing in Blosser's and Brady's classes to connect more deeply to themselves and invites those listening to expand their boundaries to include others' realities.

The section concludes with a caution from second-grade teacher Daniel Rouse, who is given a lesson on mindfulness by one of his students.

Empty Rooms, Magic Oysters, and Talking Pencils

Rebecca Martin-Scull

Silence, mindful attention, and guided visualization are helpful in many ways in lower school and middle school library and study skills classes at Media-Providence Friends School. Nearly every class starts with silence (if I forget, the kids usually remind me!) guided in various ways by a chime or the use of the small wooden drum my son made for me. My classes range from Pre-kindergarten through eighth grade, so the length of the silence varies from a few seconds between repeated striking of the chime or drum up to five minutes spaced between a beginning and an ending chime. The number of chimes or the length between two chimes increases as the year goes on and students can handle the challenge of longer periods of silence. With three-year-olds, it's especially beautiful to see their little faces with eyes and mouths closed, listening for the chime sound to fade away. This is a good way to prepare a class to hear a story or do other work, especially if they have just come in from recess. Exploring how students use the silence in these short sessions is also a good lead-in to how they might use the silence in Meeting for Worship.

Other uses for chimes and silence occur in the middle of a class. When student energy levels rise higher or sink lower than is beneficial for what we are doing, when students are experiencing a "mental block," or when they are preparing for a stressful situation such as a test, using the chimes with or without a period of silence is helpful. Most recently, in a middle school study skills course, the students experienced mental blocks about how to answer a question for a humanities assignment. We were going over a project related to the play Our Town. One instruction was to complete the following statement from the play with a paragraph about themselves: "Mama, do you know what I love most in the world, do you?" Students were to begin their paragraph by finishing the sentence, "The thing I love most in the world is ____." The students were really stumped, and some were conflicted about how to answer, especially since they felt that to answer with anything but "my parents" seemed like some kind of betrayal. So I suggested we use the chimes and silence. I instructed the students to hold the question in their minds, or better still in their hearts, and just let it be there, sit with it without trying to force an answer. I assured them I was not going to ask them to have an answer at the end of the silence, that this was just a way for them to hold the question in their awareness. This was an opportunity to practice mindfulness of the question so it could evolve for them. We spent about ten minutes in silence. Students said the silent time helped, and before the class ended, they each were able to do a written brainstorm of possible answers. Eventually, they completed the assignment successfully and on time.

Guided visualizations are useful to help students learn to look at life situations non-judgmentally. I teach students that by entering into a guided visualization, they are activating the frontal lobes of their brains. We call this section of the brain "The Boss." Such visualizations can be used to activate "The Boss" and help students develop their own sense of centeredness and safety. From this experience, students can become proactive in containing and examining strong feelings that may otherwise hijack their brains into reactivity. A favorite visualization among second-graders and older children is "The Empty Room," where they use visualization to imagine a safe space to which they can retreat when they need calm or have difficult feelings to deal with. The meditation guides them through the process of creating this safe inner space. Once there, they are guided to create a container of some kind into which they can place uncomfortable, difficult feelings when they need to take a break from them. This is different from ignoring, denying, or "stuffing" the feelings. Instead, students are guided to be aware of themselves and their feelings, take out a feeling and hold it in their hands, examine it and become aware of its shape, color, texture. They then place the feeling in a special container until the end of the meditation period. This process can be repeated with as many feelings as necessary. When the meditation period is drawing to a close, students can either choose to be done with the feeling and let it go, examine the feeling to see how it has evolved, or decide to keep the feeling in the container and revisit it later. Most students report that they enjoy going to the empty room in their minds and use this technique in a variety of settings. With their permission, I've noted three examples:

> One student imagined a paper shredder in addition to the container to hold difficult emotions. Anger and feelings he was ready to let go of he put through the shredder. If he was angry with someone and needed to talk to her about how something she had done or

said made him feel, that feeling went into the container for further decision after some rest.

Another student said upset feelings are like pieces of jelly that jiggle and have a heartbeat. When done with one, you put it in a glass jar with the others, and it slowly melts into one of the other jelly pieces. Then it's just dissolved and you feel better.

Yet another student said that her concerns were ugly when she found them, but she turned them into pearls, which eventually turned into a heart when the student was finished working on them. The student eventually put the heart back into herself by holding it on her chest where it magically reabsorbed. She said this felt fine and having it back inside her reminded her how she dealt with the original difficult feeling.

For younger students (pre-kindergarten through first grade), we use the "Magic Oyster" visualization. This much shorter process evolved out of reading the book *The Oyster's Secret* by William Barrett Morris. To do this visualization, we use some tools: the book, some real oyster shells, a string of pearls, and a jar of gritty sand. After reading the book we handle both the sand and the string of pearls. We talk about how the gritty, rough sand is what gets into the oyster and causes "oyster tears," which wrap around the sand and turn it into a pearl. Then we talk about gritty, ouchy feelings we have each had and the situations in which we had them. Finally we talk about how wonderful it would be if we could each have an imaginary, magical oyster to help us when we have ouchy feelings. Then we close our eyes and are guided to imagine how one of the ouchy feelings we have felt looks, see ourselves holding that feeling in our hand, see the magic oyster smiling at us and opening its shell so we can give it our ouchy feeling. Then we see the oyster close its shell. We rest awhile. Then the oyster smiles at us, opens its shell and we have a beautiful pearl instead of the ouchy feeling.

Guided visualization can have its pitfalls, so it is important to make sure that your students are comfortable with the idea of doing this process. There are some students who cannot visualize. All they see is blackness or a few muted colors floating, but they cannot "see" objects in their imagination. These students often use the quietness and guiding voice to listen with their eyes open, focused on an object in the room. On rare occasions, I have had a student who found such an activity profoundly uncomfortable and threatening. There was apparently no safe place in the mind. In cases like this, I talk privately with the student to find out what would be comfortable and to offer alternatives, such as quietly reading a book or drawing a picture, either in a separate part of the room or in a different room. Giving students a way to tell you if they become uncomfortable during the process and exploring comfort levels regarding visualization is an important part of developing self-awareness and helping students be effective self-advocates.

I use guided visualization to show older students the power of the brain-body connection. The students work in pairs. One partner (the subject) stretches out and gets comfortable on the floor. Once they are settled and say they are comfortable, the other partner (the data collector) takes the starting pulse rate of the subject partner and writes it down. Then we do a guided meditation. When it has ended, the data collector again checks the subject's pulse rate. Usually that rate has decreased as a result of the calming visualization. Then the partners switch places and we do the experiment again. Students are usually quite surprised at the extent to which their thoughts affect their bodies.

I've learned that these class exercises can go in unexpected directions. When they do, it is important for the teacher to be centered, mindful, and curious enough to go with what is arising. One of my favorite experiences along those lines was of this very brain-body connection exercise. At the end of the experiment a young man (the subject) looked totally relaxed, absolutely melting into the floor with a beatific smile on his face. When we checked his second pulse rate it was much higher than the starting measure. Yet when he rose from the meditation he was talking about how that was the most relaxed he had ever felt! Subsequent questioning revealed that he had been able to visualize the walk through the quiet forest, the sound of the river flowing through the forest, and the waterfall. But his creative mind had seen Native Americans with bows and arrows across the river and he had to dive into the river, swim fast, and climb up a steep bank to hide behind the waterfall. Then he relaxed just before I ended the visualization. Of course his pulse rate was up, and it was still a great example of the influence of the mind on the body!

Mindful attention, guided visualization and a sense of humor can also be used to create helpful memory aids. For example, let's say a student or class repeatedly comes to library unprepared, minus a pencil.

Have students close their eyes and see themselves in their homeroom, gathering their books and getting ready for library class. Those who are centered enough to have picked up their pencils will see their pencils smiling at them happily, feel the pencils snuggling into their hands, pockets, or book bags with a little wiggle, and hear their pencils making a happy, contented little sound. But for those who start to walk out of their room without a pencil, their pencil leaps out of their desk, and morphs to life-size, complete with arms and legs and a very loud voice. The pencil will run after them crying to them, "Please, please take me to library class!" At this point, either with happy, contented pencils, or with large upset pencils the students arrive at the library and introduce their pencils to the teacher by name. She welcomes them and class begins. When I did this with a class the number of students bringing a pencil to class the following week went from four to twelve. I was also introduced to quite a few pencils by name that week!

Nurturing the Inner Garden

Denise Aldridge

Time, silence, growth, and mindfulness: the third- and fourth-grade children of the Friends School of Atlanta embarked on a garden study in early September that led them down a deep and meaningful path. "The Edible Garden" is a small garden site between the main school building and the playground. The children pass it every day, twice a day, on the way to the playground. The garden is divided into six sections, one for each class, with grass walkways between each plot. It was established by the loving manual labor of students and parents in 2003. A soaker hose system ("the black snake") waters the garden. The study began with a simple query: Although we see the garden every day, how closely do we really look?

In the heat of early September, the garden is a riot of color, growth, and life. With initial directions of "draw what you see," the children brought a clipboard, a white piece of paper, and a pencil and walked around the garden sections. Each child was asked to carefully choose one particular plant, flower, or fruit to study. Once they had chosen their subject, the children sat for forty minutes during their science class in silence in the warm heat, studying, observing, and drawing. Each child colored his or her drawing with colored pencils and dated and titled their work. The initial drawings were stylized, simple drawings of general flowers, tomatoes, insects, and leaves. The children and teachers revisited the drawings and asked questions, such as "What shape is a flower?" "What shape is a leaf?" "Are they all the same?" "What shape is a tomato?" "What shape is a bee?" There was no right answer, which prompted more intentional study.

For the second study of the garden, the children selected either the same or a different area to focus on. In early October, the air was still warm. The children were surprised to notice that the garden was not the same garden they had studied in detail in September. They noted the changes with each other and excitedly told the teacher about new seed pods, ripe peppers and tomatoes, and flowers that are pink and orange and white and purple. They observed that the flowers of chrysanthemums open in concentric circles. The flowers of the morning glory open like a trumpet. The flowers of mint and basil are white and stand up like spikes. The leaves of basil are round, while the leaves of mint are serrated. Plus, you can pick and eat both leaves. The bees really like these flowers. The children noticed that some peppers were red and some were green. The children revisited the tomatoes, which were ripe. The yellow flowers of the tomato plants were absent, but there were small cherry tomatoes and big beefsteak tomatoes. The teacher and children revisited the drawings and asked, "Are all tomatoes red? Are they all round? Are they all the same?"

The third study of the garden began in late October. The scarecrow was out by the garden and the air was getting cool. The children came out with determination to find their spot and "their" plants. In the silence and coolness, the children noted there was less "music" from the bugs and birds. There were fewer bees. They observed that the garden in the fall is different than in the late summer. They wanted to study the tomatoes. They discovered that not all tomatoes are red. They observed that tomatoes are not always round or perfect "like at the store." They began including the blemishes, bumps, and ovals in their drawings. They included the green of unripeness, the brownish red of rot, and the black spots. They noticed that the rotten ones on the ground made nice homes for insects. The tomato vines, in particular, were studied. They twist and turn, and, the children discovered, they are hairy. Why would a vine have hair? Did we include the hair in the drawing? There were no yellow flowers on the vines at this time of year. The basil and mint had lost their flowers and a lot of their leaves. The broccoli was showing signs of becoming food for bugs and the strawberry plants had gone dormant. The mustard was quite large, though, and many children began to study lettuce. They found that lettuce leaves come in all shapes and sizes—divided, serrated, smooth and round, short and spiky, with the baby leaves on the inside and the older, bigger leaves on the outside. The children noticed that plants have veins "just like us!" On the underside of many leaves, the children found egg sacs and cocoons. The children spent time coloring their drawings and reflecting on what they observed. Inside the classroom, the drawings were revisited and discussed. As children looked at each other's work, they realized they were each looking at the garden differently. The drawings were big and finely detailed.

Doing their garden study, the children learned to stop and look for a long time at one thing. In the stillness and silence, the children opened themselves up to the life that surrounded them. They found that "You have to be very silent. When I am being silent, I am just listening to the wind blowing and looking at the plants. I just feel free." The children learned to see where leaves attach and that every leaf is different and "some vines have spikes and some don't." The children observed that "All the tomatoes aren't the same color and the only time they change is when they grow, go rotten, or when a bug eats them." While sitting in stillness in the hot sun of September through the cool wind of October, they found life and death, growth and variety, and each child "learned to draw just what I see…to draw with brilliance." In sharing the garden-study drawings, the children shared their perspective of the garden with other students and teachers. "I liked looking at the plants and animals. It made me feel wonderful. I want the whole world to do what we did!" The children took what they learned from the garden study and applied it to subsequent field trips during the year, studying the pond and the goat farm in detail as well as studying the animals in the classroom with greater concentration. In quiet stillness, one can observe the many differences that make up the environment and "Your mind is sharper and you realize things more quickly, like a plant has a new color tomato or…the vines are different shades and a potato has another sprout."

The children reflected on how drawing and studying the garden affected them and made them mindfully aware of how "the garden is like life." "When I observe the garden, I feel like I am floating." "The garden is peaceful and quiet. The garden is a place of hidden power. The gardens grow beautiful things." The children look forward to studying the garden in the spring because "when you walk through the garden, you feel your inner light." Already the potatoes and bulbs inside our classroom have started to sprout. The children anticipate the garden study because "Walking in the garden is like walking with God…like walking on a cloud."

Currently, we have begun a project designing a square-foot garden, where the children can grow plants that they can study further—and even eat. Many different parts make up a vibrant, living, healthy garden. We extended this concept to ourselves and our class, noticing that we are all different and we all contribute to a healthy, vibrant, active class and community. We are all growing and changing. No one is the same from month to month or year to year. We all are together in our classroom environment, our school, our community, our nation, and our world. This poem from one of the children provides a lyrical summary for the composite experience in studying the garden:

I learned…
Not all vines are green
Not all tomatoes are red
Not all peppers are always red
There are lots of different kinds of flowers
Not all vegetables are perfect—like at the store.

Writing Is an Act of Love:
Mindfulness and Micro-fiction

Hope Blosser

The paradox of mindfulness is to find the luminosity in our mundane experiences. There is no magic trick here, no mantra to dissolve our worries and foster peace of mind. The only tool mindfulness offers is to pay close attention to life as it presents itself. Without judgment or criticism, mindfulness calls on us to acknowledge what arises and become comfortable with emotions and attitudes we usually don't want to own up to. Only when we let go of our desire to run away from these emotions and allow ourselves to become immersed in our hurt, anger, or embarrassment are we finally able to connect with the fluidity and universality of such emotions. This process, in turn, helps loosen our grip on the perceived permanence of our separate identities and create a space for healing and connection rather than division, for laughter and celebration instead of judgment and criticism.

As a Zen practitioner and English teacher, I am often asked how I integrate the practice of mindfulness in my middle-school classes. These questions move and excite me, but all too often the constant demands of the classroom would wear down my initial inspiration, and carving out time for reflection got squeezed out of an already cluttered curriculum. I was delighted to find a perfect opportunity to practice mindfulness in the classroom while preparing to teach *The House on Mango Street* by Sandra Cisneros. While telling about the process of writing her first novel, Cisneros explained how she found herself "exchanging shame for celebration." That simple phrase from her introduction reminded me of the transformative powers of mindfulness and helped me find a place within the existing curriculum to combine academic objectives with meditative insights. This essay attempts to capture how the practice of mindfulness is the ideal complement to the study of the micro-fiction genre.

Methodology

The unit begins by listening to an audio version of Sandra Cisneros's introduction as a whole class. Twelve- and thirteen-year-old students listen while Cisneros explains the search she undertook as a young woman to uncover her own voice, a voice unlike that of the mostly white, male European authors she was studying. She describes feeling different and separate from her peers and deciding to write with a voice that reflected the neighborhoods she came from. When the phrase "exchanging shame for celebration" is read aloud, I copy it on the board, along with St. Francis's famous adage, "If you bring forth that which is within you, that which is within you will save you. If you do not bring forth that which is within you, that which is within you will destroy you."

Once the introduction is finished, the students are usually looking more awake and inspired, and we focus our attention on the two quotes. I ask the students to sit in small groups and discuss what each passage means to them. Then we share our answers as a whole class. I ask them to consider what it means to celebrate the parts of ourselves that may usually be hidden by shame, self-hatred, or a sense of separateness, what it would look and feel like to put into words the very stories we try to ignore. I emphasize that the process Cisneros and St. Francis both point to takes great courage and fearlessness, but that telling the honest stories of our lives creates a freedom from the same emotions that long to keep them hidden.

Even the orneriest middle-school students are generally pretty inspired at this point—they are so drawn to authentic communication with adults—and I ask them to write their first micro-fiction story. We don't discuss the numerous conventions and tools they will be asked to apply to their work later; instead, I read the title piece from Cisneros's book *The House on Mango Street* aloud, and the students craft their own pieces about where they live. At the end of the first class, students share their work and exchange feedback. Starting the unit with an extended period of listening to Cisneros's language, followed by time for independent writing and sharing with others, fosters a sense of enthusiasm and ownership that will support all of our work to come.

The instruction I give on peer feedback is one of the initial steps to mindfulness, and it guides students to a place of attentiveness. The rules for feedback are few: students should avoid giving vague praise such as, "I really liked it! It was very good!" or, alternatively, "I just couldn't get into that piece." Instead, I ask them to pay attention to the exact words and phrases they remember after the reader has finished. Those words are the strongest, most alive parts of the writing, and the more specific the praise, the better equipped each writer feels about creating successful pieces in the future. This process of paying close attention to one another's language also helps establish a community of writers who feel empowered to take the risks needed to create vignettes that truly reflect the reality of their lives and learn from one another instead of simply fulfilling the requirements dictated by their teachers. If, by the end of the first day, most of the kids' faces show a combination of relief and pride, it has been a great success.

After several days using this method, we begin to look at Cisneros's writing with a more critical eye. Since students have been reading sections of the book at home and are more familiar with the author's style at this point, I ask them what patterns they notice in the vignettes. Several responses erupt at once. "They're soooo short!" someone booms. I translate this observation into the word "micro-fiction," and write it on the board as one of Cisneros's writing tools. Other tools are volunteered, including the use of figurative language, simple vocabulary and syntax, the lack of quotation marks to denote dialogue, and unusual details. I add to this list a couple more tools, including the use of a powerful, authoritative voice and a tool that can only be described as "what she says by not saying it." The students immediately understand the sense of spaciousness I'm targeting with this tool, and we look for examples where Cisneros creates a scene and leaves out certain details so that the reader is left with a sense of mysterious possibility, as in the following excerpt in which Cisneros describes how her main character feels when a teacher passing by sees her in front of her house:

> You live *there?*
> *There.* I had to look to where she pointed – the third floor, the paint peeling, wooden bars Papa nailed on the windows so we wouldn't fall out. You live there? The way she said it made me feel like nothing. *There.* I lived *there.* I nodded.
> I knew then I had to have a house. A real house. One I could point to.

After the students have copied down these tools I introduce the micro-fiction portfolio assignment, explaining that each student will be required to submit seven to nine typed pages of stories about their own lives. Once the initial shock wears off, we create a topics list, which will help students maintain their momentum and keep them from running out of ideas. We turn to Cisneros's book as a model, and students pick out the following topics: family, friends, physical traits (like hair or toes or belly buttons), first experiences (like jobs or dances or dates), people we love, neighbors, the unspoken rules of certain groups or places, rumors about people in the neighborhood, stories passed down in the family, and many more.

For the next week and a half, students are given time to draft pieces in class. I require that they experiment with each of the tools we went over and include as many topics from our list as fit into their own lives. I remind students to provide a quiet, contemplative space for one another so that they are able to find the stories they want or may need to tell. Many students get to work immediately and write for the entire time; others may add to or review their topics list before drafting. When students get stuck, as they inevitably do, I act as a troubleshooter by helping them to uncover the story that may be buried within a piece or to abandon a lifeless piece and move on to another topic altogether. In order to maintain a sense of mindfulness, I ask my students simple questions such as, "What is the most important part of this piece?" or "What tools do you think work best here?" and listen attentively to their responses before adding any of my suggestions. Listening in this way keeps me, as the instructor, from falling into the habit of telling the student what to do or where to go with a story. This method benefits the students as well by bolstering their sense of ownership over their lives and experiences and compelling each of them to grapple with the process of expressing themselves clearly and concisely.

Celebrations

On the last day of the unit each student takes a turn reading one vignette aloud to their peers. We practice giving specific, focused feedback and applaud each person's efforts. As their instructor, I sit back at the end of the day, completely blown away by the depth of the emotions they reveal so willingly and the deep humanity and compassion these early adolescents deliver to the page time and time again. By following the simple instructions of paying attention to what happens in their lives, each student submits pieces that are part prose and part poetry, painful and uplifting, honest and mysterious. Some students confess times when they were not their "best" selves—one of the topics I asked them to add to their topics list. In one example, a student investigates the numerous emotions beneath her desire to tease a younger cousin:

> I don't know why I was so mean to Gabi. Maybe it was because I was jealous that she was spoiled. Maybe it's because I felt like my sister loved Gabi more than me. Maybe it was because she stole my

spotlight. Maybe it was because we weren't very mature. Maybe it was because we were so alike and stubborn that we couldn't get along. Before she was born, I got all the attention, and I was the one that the adults paid attention to because I was the youngest.

By honestly investigating and stating the conflicting emotions, the author feels compassion for herself in this individual act, and it broadens to become an experience everyone can relate to and sympathize with. The author's individual shame and regret is transformed into forgiveness and self-acceptance.

Writers also address times when they feel afraid and victimized. In the next example, a young woman delves into the everyday experience of taking mass transit:

The subway is a very scary place for me. Every time I get on a train, there's always at least one male who looks at me. I don't know why they look at me. I'm not pretty. Sometimes, I think that they are looking at my chest or other places that they aren't supposed to look at, and it makes me uncomfortable. Why are they looking at me? I want to ask them sometimes. I don't like them looking at me the way they do. Sometimes, it's teenage boys who look at me. Around fourteen to sixteen years old. But usually, it's adult men looking at me. Around twenty-two years old and older. Stop! Stop looking at me! I want to yell. Just go away! I get off the train and start walking home. Tomorrow. Tomorrow will be better, I think to myself. But, of course, it isn't any better. It's always the same or worse. I give up. I surrender. I'll just deal with their looks since that's the only thing I can do.

Even though the author claims to have to put up with the men's unwanted attention, the act of writing so honestly about the experience opens up a space for the impassioned observer in her and reduces her sense of helpless victimization. She may not be able to step up to her aggressors in person, but she has voiced her outrage on the page and, in doing so, released herself from their power and the likelihood of feeling the same way in the future.

Another topic each student is asked to include is what I classify as "The Forgotten and Overlooked Ones." Students are instructed to consider writing as an act of love, just like the act of turning one's attention toward, rather than away from, a needy face or an outstretched hand.

The practice of mindful attention and suspended judgment appears in the form of pieces dedicated to homeless people, fruit vendors on the local corner, and other people who are a part of our daily lives but rarely honored with our attention. In the following excerpt, a young writer turns her attention toward those she tends to ignore and, by earnestly probing the depths of her emotions, describes what she would like to do for the homeless and lonely people in her neighborhood:

> When I walk down to the train station, I see an older lady, with a tiny sweater on and old sneakers, and she doesn't look very warm in this thirty-degree weather. She makes me upset. I run down the stairs, not paying attention to her question. Spare change, miss? No. I have nothing for you.

> I know how to make soup. Tomato soup. Vegetable soup. Chicken noodle is my best yet....It's such a warm and welcoming food. Its light steam and salty taste are good for this weather. And the homeless ones I always see.

> I know what it feels like. To be so cold you feel like your toes will fall off. And to be lonely. To have to sit alone in an unfamiliar place. To be scared. To feel like no one cared. To be said no to. No. Warmth is all we need. The homeless and I. So what I'll do is give them the warmth they need. The warmth any soup can give. The warmth I can give.

Difficult interactions with parents and peers—such pressing topics for middle-school students—are also investigated and processed. In this piece, a young woman thoughtfully investigates her reasons for going against her own desires:

> In my whole life only one person has ever asked me out on a date. I was the first of my group of friends to be asked out. They all made a very big deal about it. Not just my friends, but the whole grade....Even though not a lot of people liked him, I still wanted to say yes. But I could not. I could not, because everyone was telling me to say no. I could not, because, if I did, everyone would make fun of me for going out with him....The day I said no to him, I went straight home after school....While I was in the shower I burst into tears....I want him to ask me out again so that I can say yes, and re-bandage his heart....If I could tell him one thing why I said no, it would be that it was peer pressure, not that I did not like you.

The next author describes in brutally honest detail her interactions with her mother:

> I get twenty dollars every month because I don't have a Papi anymore. He and mother needed a break. I don't have a Mami either sometimes. She is my mother. I don't want a mother. She gave me a life. One I did not ask for. One she says I spend being lazy....Why don't you help with the dishes? Why don't you offer help? Why are you giving me an attitude?...What is wrong with you, Bianca? What is wrong with you?

Being mindful doesn't always have to mean writing about difficult or painful times. The playful nature of mindfulness leads many students to take up lighter topics, like the completion of the portfolio itself, as in the following example:

> Two weeks ago, I was assigned a project called the micro-fiction portfolio. We had to write seven to nine pages of vignettes in the style of Sandra Cisneros....We began drafting these stories in English class....I had written all my vignettes....I thought that typing and revising would be the easy part. It is now 11:10 on Sunday night, December 16th. My portfolio is due tomorrow. I am tired and cold. The thing that I want to do most right now is just go to sleep, but no, I cannot do that because I have to finish this report that my teacher assigned weeks ago, but me being me, I had to leave to the very last second to finish. Good night.

Conclusions

At the end of his life, the Buddha's last message to his devotees was that each person must find his or her own light to guide them, instead of depending on someone or something else to rely on. The Buddha encouraged self-reliance through compassion and wisdom of self. Buddhists all over the world practice mindfulness as a way of waking up to that self within that does not need to be improved upon or altered in any way.

Although *The House on Mango Street* unit may not expose students to the challenging vocabulary and complex sentence structure that will help prepare them for future assignments, the simple language and straightforward description of difficult emotions used so lovingly by Sandra Cisneros calls out to young readers. The practice of mindfulness helps writers look within themselves and find their own unique voice. These voices may be one of the most valuable gifts we as educators can offer our students. The messages these voices offer may also contribute to a broader definition of academic success, one that doesn't overlook the need for compassion for oneself and others.

"Why Are We Doing This?"
Nurturing Academic Mindfulness
Through Self-Grading

Douglas Tsoi

"Teacher, why are we doing this?" All of us have been asked this
question by a student at some point. When I first started teaching, the
question threatened and angered me. *Because I'm the teacher* was what
I felt like saying and was probably behind whatever answer I actually
gave. After a while, I came to realize that this was *the* essential question
for students. "Why are we doing this?" was deep wisdom bubbling to
the surface; it was a student asking for, demanding, purposeful activity.

So many of our students go to school uncritically. They go to school
because they are expected to. They go to school because they've never
known anything else. They study to receive the praise of parents and
teachers by getting good grades. Or at the high school level they've
internalized that motivation enough to say they try to get good grades.
When asked why they want to get good grades, they answer to get into
a "good college." When asked why they want to get into a good college,
they answer so that they can "be successful." Some are more honest and
say that they want to be rich.

I see two problems with students studying to get good grades to get
into a good college to be successful. First, it causes students to study
for some ineffable future and not remain fully present in the classroom.
They become unmindful to the deeper purposes of learning. Second,
because they are taught the importance of their transcripts for college
admissions, it causes students to focus on the *symbols* of learning—
grades—not the learning itself.

A Quaker high school and a progressive education should offer more
than that. Our students should know the reason their education is
important, why what they are doing, the lessons, the skills, and the
practices we teach are important in and of themselves. If one of our
core values is being present, the high school education we offer needs
to be about high school, not preparing for college. Our students should
care passionately about what they are learning because what they are

learning is vital to their present lives, touches greater questions they care about, and feeds their souls.

In the spring terms of 2005 and 2006, I ran the following lesson plan for my ninth-grade social studies class to deepen the students' self-awareness as learners. I wanted them to think deeply about the academic pressures around them and how these pressures affected their motivation to learn. I wanted my students to explore the meaning of grades, of academic integrity, and of community.

The lesson plan began when I handed out the following proposal and asked students if they would learn more if they graded themselves for the third term. Then, in a Meeting for Worship for Business, each class came to unity on whether they wanted the responsibility.

A Proposal for Self-Determination

Should students decide how they want to learn and how they want to be evaluated? Should students in this class grade themselves? Would self-grading increase or decrease learning? Here are a few queries to think about:

1. Are grades given or earned?
2. What are the purposes of having grades?
3. Who should decide how well a student has learned something— the student or the teacher?
4. What does it mean to "learn" something?
5. Would you work more or less if (a) no grades in this class were given, or (b) you gave yourself the grade?
6. Should course grading account for different types of learners?
7. Should assignments and classroom activities account for different types of learners?
8. How do you build a system that rewards hard workers? Is hard work the only thing you should grade?
9. What is academic "success"? Who gets to decide if you were successful—the teacher or student?
10. Why are you at school? Do you really want to be here? Why?

11. How does competition affect your learning and your perception of how much you learned?

12. How does being graded affect your learning and your perception of how much you learned?

13. If students could determine their own grade, would academic integrity be maintained?

14. If students could determine their own grade, how would other students' self-evaluations affect how you would feel about the self-grading system"?

My hope is that the conversation that emerges from these queries, particularly the last two questions, introduces issues like fairness, purpose, academic community, integrity, self-determination versus totalitarianism, and dependence. Are 15-year-olds old enough to handle deciding if they should get homework and what grades they should get? Is a teacher's job to provide, to the best of his or her ability, some "objective" measure of academic success? Would students have learned as much this year if I wasn't a demanding teacher? If not, is it damaging that I play on their natural desire to please and to succeed?

I had incorporated silence in every class and taught through Socratic dialogue. All year, the classroom was set up in a circle so that students were conditioned to look at and listen to each other, not the teacher. I handed out a pamphlet on Quaker Meeting for Business, discussed the role of a clerk, and chose a clerk for the first day.

In the week of business meeting that followed, each class used the Quaker decision-making process to come to unity on adopting self-grading, but only after tackling such issues as how one learns and how others learn, what is evidence of learning, and why one feels motivated to learn. For some, the proposal was threatening: they were doing well and did not want change; for them, grading themselves stripped the grade of its objective meaning. For others, the proposal was an opportunity and a test: they wanted to see if they could handle the responsibility to continue learning without an adult evaluating them, but they were afraid that they wouldn't have the discipline. For still others— students who were working hard but whose test scores and papers were not meeting my highest standards—the proposal meant that they could give themselves the grade they felt they "deserved."

Overlying all those issues were concerns students had that they couldn't trust themselves, or each other, to give themselves honest grades. They had to struggle with problems about grading in a diverse academic community. What *should* grades quantify: performance or effort? The answer either way would justify some and threaten others. Students asked me during the Meeting for Business whether I would be upset if someone who "clearly didn't deserve" an A gave themselves an A. I responded that normally students are subject to the teacher; by proposing this grading system, I wanted them to be subject to themselves. I told them that I suspected that anyone who gave themselves a grade they felt they didn't earn would one day remember it—one year, five years, or twenty years from now—and their conscience would be pricked, which would be a far more important lesson in integrity than anything I could do in the class. Beyond that, I contributed little; the conversations were deep and enriching enough without me. In the end, I think the classes decided to self-grade because it felt important. Because grades hold such a sway at an independent school, self-grading meant they could take values that they were being taught at the school, values like integrity, community, and equality, and see if they could take the responsibility to live them. Self-grading let them practice Quaker values deeply, personally, and meaningfully.

For the rest of the term, students completed their homework in preparation for the next day, but I did not check it. At the end of the year, they completed take-home finals and we corrected them together in class, each student grading his or her own test. They then wrote self-evaluations and gave themselves a grade for the third term (which was averaged with their previous terms' grades for a final year-long grade). The first year, my students wrote their own evaluations, which I typed into their report card. The second year, after a master teacher suggested it was my professional obligation to provide feedback, I added a paragraph of evaluation after the students'. The move was a good one; my evaluation gave the student and his or her parent an independent assessment of the student's performance, which was especially important if it did not mirror the student's self-perception.

Did self-grading nurture mindfulness and mindful learning? Was it is vital to the students' lives, did it touch greater questions they care about and feed their souls? Did it inculcate the values we teach at a Quaker school? Now, two or three years later, I emailed my former students asking what they remembered of the lesson plan. Here are some their responses.

Grading myself was really difficult actually because I knew I wasn't working as hard as I should have been. Looking back, I regret not reading the material some nights and not getting the full benefit of your class. One of the reasons I think I started doing better in school is because of your class. When I was being graded, it felt like it wasn't my fault if I got a bad grade because I usually don't do badly in school—it was just your class. I had someone else to blame—you. I used the excuse that it didn't matter if I worked harder because I'd probably just get the same grade. But when third term came and I knew I'd be grading myself, I felt bad for not doing my work. I remember actually reading the third term of your class because I had to prove to *myself, not you,* that I learned something, not you.

I remember trying to reach a decision as to if we should use the "give yourself a grade" system through a Quakerly consensus. I felt like it was hard for everyone to reach a clear-cut decision. At first it seemed like the choice was clear, who wouldn't want to give themselves their own grade? However, as we talked about this some more we realized that we might be inclined just to give ourselves a grade that didn't reflect the work we had done. This thought led me to the question of "What's the importance of a grade anyway?" Why does it matter that the grade reflects our work? That question itself, though, is important as it relates to honesty and truth, specifically self-honesty. Also, I learned that good group decision-making requires more in-depth thinking as opposed to just absorbing what's being said without fully questioning it to understand it better. Example: All of us were listening to what was being said, but we didn't make any progress until we tried understanding where everyone was coming from and then talking about that, so that we had a broader/fuller understanding.

Even coming from a Quaker school previously, it seemed so strange to have to evaluate myself entirely. I had always had to do self-evaluation type exercises but I had never been trusted with something as important as my grade, and it was the first time that I really felt pressure to come up with my own opinion about myself as a student. But after having to go through (the self-grading exercise) I feel like it has been much easier to know the amount of effort that I put into something, not only in classes but in other things like sports. I remember that I gave myself a B+ and it was so hard to make that decision with integrity. I'm not proud of the grade that I gave myself, because I realize now that I could have tried much harder but as a freshman I wasn't really aware of that. It was a valuable lesson to learn, especially as early as fourteen years old. The week-long Meeting for Business or what I remember of it was pretty chaotic. But the fact that it was a week long says a lot. It showed that one person can make a decision quickly based on just one fact, but in a group setting it's much better to come to the right decision, because almost every piece of information and opinion was covered and discussed.

The exercise helped nurture mindfulness because I finally realized that my education was more than just a letter grade with a teacher evaluating me every step of the way. I had to think about how well I had done in the class for myself and with that I was able to understand that my education was for myself and no one else and that I should continue learning with that in my mind and to always do the best I can, not for other people but for me.

When you first gave us the assignment, I remember thinking to myself, "I'm not going to give myself an A, because I want Douglas to respect me," because I really looked up to you. During the week-long process however, I did do a lot of self-reflecting. I took into account the quality of my work, as well as the subject matter and substance. Most important to me, though, was the effort I put into my work. I ended up giving myself a B+ and thought that was fair. I wasn't upset with others who I knew gave themselves As, because I was happy knowing I came to my decision through intense thought. I was content with my B+ and my integrity.

I definitely learned a lot about my motivations. Prior to the exercise, I believed the pressure on me to do well came from others and that I had a certain image to uphold. I learned that my motivation came mostly from within me. Not only was it my competitive nature, but a personal standard that I myself felt I had to meet. Had I been caught up in what others thought of me, I think I would have given myself the A, you know, to appease my parents and everyone else that looked at my report card. I learned that I worked hard for me, and to this day I believe that is most important. I'm not doing this for anyone else. Sure, I'd like to make my parents and teachers proud, but not if I'm not getting anything out of it. This is my education, and it's up to me to make something of it.

The thing that strikes me most about the students' responses is how much students wrote about integrity. I believe that students yearn for opportunities to test themselves and their character, and this exercise was deeply meaningful for so many because it tested them. Two stories illuminate this point further. I had a student who struggled entering George School and earned a D in my class the first term. By sheer hard work and completing every extra-credit assignment, she was in a position to get an A- for the course if she gave herself an A for the third term. After grading her final exam (which I never saw but on which she told me she made critical mistakes), she gave herself a B, thus earning a B+ for the course. She says that she is proudest of that B+ of all her grades in high school. The second story is of an extremely talented student who also was in the position to get an A- for the course if she would give herself an A for the third term. But knowing that she did not work as hard that third term because I did not grade her, she gave herself a B, again earning a B+ for the course. It was her only non-A grade on her transcript for her first two years and she says that she is prouder of that B+ than all her As.

I've had many students say that the process our class went through around self-grading was one of the most meaningful experiences of their high school education. Having chosen to evaluate themselves, they had to confront issues of motivation, independence, self-advocacy, and integrity in themselves and ask themselves what, and who, their educations were really for. They had to ask themselves why they were doing what they were doing and they had to struggle with the complexity of the answer. My hope is that by asking themselves these questions as high school freshmen, they will be more likely to keep asking them for the rest of their lives.

Making Sand Mandalas:
An Exercise in Impermanence and Letting Go

Eric Mayer

A silver bird
flies over the autumn lake.
When it has passed,
the lake's surface does not try
to hold on to the image of the bird.

— Buddhist master Huong Hai

The monks couldn't come. After several weeks of phone calls to a group of traveling Tibetan monks, I gave up on the possibility that they would come to our high school to publicly build a sand mandala. I had invited them as part of our study of Buddhism. A sand mandala—which is painstakingly built and then summarily swept into a jar and poured into a stream—seemed the perfect expression of the Buddhist principles of impermanence and non-attachment. A *mandala,* from the Sanskrit meaning circle or container, is a physical meditation aid composed in a highly detailed geometric pattern. Sand mandalas are built on a template on the floor, and may range from several feet across to filling an entire room. For some Buddhists, mandalas represent the dwelling place of Buddha or another figure of focused meditation. Creating sand mandalas have been cloistered observances within Tibetan Buddhism for centuries. In the 1980s their public construction was first allowed by the Dalai Lama. Western audiences have been stupefied ever since. Incredible artistry, training, and concentration are brought to bear on a public work of art that is then destroyed in the time it takes to brush one's teeth.

Feeling dejected about the monks' non-appearance at our school, I set about a new course: could the students make sand mandalas instead? Five years later, I can't imagine doing it any other way. Although the monks would have offered ritual and grandeur, the personal experience for the students has been unrivaled in promoting growth and awareness about the fundamental nature of reality.

Borrowing from Buddhism

I am not Buddhist, nor are most of my students in our required junior-year world religions class at Westtown School, a coeducational Quaker day and boarding program in Pennsylvania. However, as we explore other religious and moral traditions, I have been guided by the Dalai Lama's advice that we ought to borrow from his tradition and return to our own. While I am sensitive to issues of cultural misappropriation, a sincere approach to borrowing from Buddhism has felt both respectful and useful.

Making a Mandala

Students work in groups of four to build a sand mandala as the concluding exercise to our unit on Buddhism. Mandalas must be made of sand or other granular material (sugar, salt, soil), and should be based on the pattern of a historic mandala. Sand is crucial because it represents matter in its most elemental and dissolved form; anything more permanent weakens the exercise.

Given the complexity and detail of the Tibetan mandalas, I advise students to simplify their pattern while retaining overall geometry and proportion. I am also clear that they should strive for beauty; the finished mandala should be exquisite to behold. Students are to work in "noble silence," using tools that they fashion—usually from straws, plastic bags, and silverware. Noble silence is a perspective that recognizes the fullness contained in silence. As in Quakerism, silence is understood as fecund. Silence is not empty; rather, it is a mode both of repose and of listening. In a world saturated with sensory stimulation, noble silence is an invitation to travel an ancient and revelatory landscape. The project takes five to ten person-hours, at which point each group presents the mandala it has created to the class.

Students are often surprised by the assignment. Many don't know what to make of its presence in a rigorous academic course. One student captured the feeling this way:

> At first the words that went through my head when Teacher Eric gave this assignment were, "This is the stupidest thing he has ever proposed that we do."

Once they get down to work, the building process often turns into something of a meditation:

> The construction of the mandala, like sawing a board, drew in my complete focus. What started as something like a game ended by being extraordinarily important. Nothing existed but the sand, me, and the project. Even my classmates seemed to disappear in the moment.

Many students articulate a soothing quality in the work:

> While building the mandala, I felt a peculiar calmness. The activity put me at ease. I was becoming aware of a childhood activity that I had long forgotten.

Some have unusual experiences:

> For some reason, the placement of the sand put me in touch with the memory of a deceased family member. The grains of sand represented all the things we had shared....The presence and later loss of the sand showed me that people and things live on in our minds, even when they are gone.

Dissolving the Mandala

The most important part of the project is the conclusion—a singularly bizarre act in a society that seeks to preserve, insure, and otherwise enshrine things of beauty. Once the students complete the mandala, they must consider, as a group, whether they are able to "liberate" it. Liberating the mandala means returning it to the earth, usually in our campus lake or a field (some have used the glen where they will one day graduate). Some groups are emotionally unable to complete this step, which creates an opportunity for learning. Either way, they write an essay about the experience. Most students have an experience similar to this one:

> It was very hard for me to liberate the mandala. I really liked how it looked, and I put in a lot of time to finish it. I better understand the idea of impermanence, but I still wish we could have kept it.

Another student described how awareness of the conclusion shaped the process:

> The knowledge that I would soon destroy the mandala gave me a sense of relief while I was making it. It allowed me to focus on my activity in the current moment, without wondering how my present action would look to me years from now. It would never become a memento.

Still others express a range of responses to the dissolution process, illustrated by these different voices:

> We dissolved our mandala in the lawn of our freshman dormitory—a place close to our hearts, but one we also had to let go as we grew. Now our mandala will be soil for the new flowers that grow there.

> When we let our work blow away on the Girls' End porch, I knew I was celebrating impermanence. Surprisingly, it was not a painful experience. I felt that the dissolving increased the value of my work. Since it doesn't exist in one place now, it exists everywhere. This is what differentiates dissolution from destruction.

> I didn't feel any regret as I ruined the mandala. If anything, I felt a little bit of happiness that I can't explain.

One winter the lesson emerged in an unpredictable way. Thinking the mandala was somehow a mess on the floor, a housekeeper at the school vacuumed it up just hours before it was due. The students were devastated. At first, I was upset, too—but then I realized how perfectly appropriate this was as a conclusion to the assignment. The vanished mandala was abrupt and startling, but it represented impermanence in all its power, and the loss of control that it can elicit.

Why This Exercise Matters

Students overwhelmingly appreciate this exercise. It is a direct and immediate experience of impermanence, creating an indelible impression of this concept so central to Buddhism. It has also been a powerful lesson in non-attachment. If impermanence characterizes life for all of us, then attachment to permanence usually brings suffering—and, hence, non-attachment emerges as the most sensible and compassionate response. Many students have written about parallels in their own lives—the need to let go, to release, to surrender. On the struggles of accepting impermanence, a student commented,

> I am wary of impermanence because I have lost someone close to me, and the pain of that loss has never left me. Sometimes, I wonder if there is any reason in building relationships when you know that the relationship is only temporary....The mandala forced me to face this question in a less personal way.

Students are sometimes enriched by making connections to other parts of our culture. The Ash Wednesday prayer is one example: "Remember that you are dust, and to dust you shall return." I often describe the Tibetan Sky Burial, in which Tibetan monks ritually offer the dead villagers to resident vultures in a final act of generosity. In several class discussions, the Crucifixion has emerged as a radical act of letting go.

Sooner or later, someone mentions that the sand mandala is an analog to our own lifespan: we strive to create a beautiful life, exercising great care and devotion, and at some point our life returns to dust and is scattered into the wind. Western pop culture tends to view this perspective as maudlin, but I have found a surprising vitality and hunger as it is considered by students. Somehow, they have connected with a deeper wisdom that seems to derive from an awareness of things *as they are*, not as we want them to be. I am reminded of the Zen proverb, "My barn having burned to the ground, I can now see the moon."

Turning Toward the Other:
Lectio Divina

Richard Brady

When I was first introduced to the Benedictine practice of prayer and scriptural reading, *lectio divina*, or "holy reading," by Mary Rose O'Reilly at a contemplative education workshop, I experienced firsthand how deeply one might connect with a small portion of text examined with another person. Reading in this mindful way is slow and measured. Few students would find it an appropriate method for reading textbooks or novels. Yet when employed as a means of encountering a poem or a short passage with depth, it can transform the reader. The following is O'Reilly's decription of *lectio* and how she has presented it to her college students:

> *Lectio divina* ("holy reading") is an ancient way of reading scripture, passed on in the Benedictine tradition. It calls us to ponder and sit with a short text until we "take it in"—a wonderful phrase contradicted by so much college reading that demands the "coverage model." As Kathleen Norris has written in *The Cloister Walk*, it is a type of reading in which "one does not try to 'cover' a certain amount of material so much as surrender to whatever word or phrase catches the attention. . . . *Lectio* respects the power of words to resonate with the full range of human experience."

In adapting *lectio* to the reading of college texts, my premise is that these readings are the product of some one's spiritual life, and they deserve the kind of attentive reading we might offer a friend who has pondered long over what he or she has to tell us.

Method — Solo exercise:
1. Center yourself in your body, mind and purpose.
2. Read the passage reflectively several times.
3. Consider the questions: What speaks to me most profoundly here? What do I feel called to "take in"? Is there something that pushes me away? Is there something I want to comment on, bring into dialogue with my own experience?
4. Write for five or ten minutes.

Method — Group exercise:
1. Keep a few minutes silence together.
2. In groups of four to six, one reads aloud while the others listen.
3. Each speaks to something the reading sparks in him or her.
4. General discussion.

When one experiences relating to a poem or passage in this way, one understands what it means to make it one's own. I suspect that the periodic use of this method might, over time, begin to affect the ways in which other reading is done, slowing it down, revealing more connections, raising more questions, making note-taking a more personal process. Teaching high school mathematics, I didn't feel it was appropriate to use *lectio* in my classes. However, I use it regularly in my workshops with educators and parents.

I frequently end these workshops with a series of meditations. For the first meditation, participants spend five minutes contemplating a poem or short passage, just hanging out with it, perhaps dwelling on a particular line or image and seeing what arises in them in response. Then I ask the participants to take another five minutes to record continuously whatever is coming up for them. Finally, I ask them to pair up with someone they don't know well or, if possible, don't know at all. Each member of the pair is given four minutes to share anything that he or she wishes about his or her experience of the reading or writing. The person listening is asked just to listen, not comment, not ask questions, say nothing, and not express approval or disapproval in any way nonverbally. Listeners can find these instructions difficult to follow. Whether their experiences were similar to or very different from their partner's, many find it hard to contain their reactions. They're not just listening to their partner but thinking about what they're hearing, comparing it to their experience, often appreciating some aspect of the sharing, occasionally having some kind of negative response. Because they're not just listening to understand but also having personal responses, their positive and negative judgments are hard to contain. In addition, because they're filtering what they're hearing through their judgment, they may not really be hearing what's being said. Some participants also find it hard to share without getting feedback. They want affirmation, want to feel that the listener not only understands but appreciates what they're sharing. And if the listener doesn't appreciate it, they'd like to know that as well so that they might clarify what they're sharing, or perhaps head in a different direction.

At the conclusion of this practice, I've been asked what the point is of withholding judgment. As teachers and parents, don't we want to let our students and children know when we're pleased or displeased with what they're saying? What is the point of just listening? I respond by saying that there are certainly situations that call for judgment. But we want to hear young people clearly. Furthermore, how are young people ever to discover and own their own feelings if they are constantly being critiqued by adults. Given a steady dose of judgment, it's all too likely that a young person will respond by becoming a pleaser or a rebel, not a person who knows and shares him or herself. More often speakers have shared how moving and rare it is to be listened to so deeply. At times the listener seems to draw forth speech by the quality of his or her attention.

The degree to which participants find the readings evocative is key factor in the activity. In presenting the *lectio divina* activity, O'Reilly gave us three passages to read, asking each participant to choose one to focus on. I also like to offer participants a choice of readings, selecting them for variety and with the particular group in mind. On more than one occasion, I've seen participants wipe away tears as they contemplated a reading. Of course, it helps to include light readings as well. Here are three of the readings I often present.

> Mulla Nasrudin (a classic Persian jokester/folk character, protagonist of many teaching stories in the Sufi tradition) decided to start a flower garden. He prepared the soil and planted the seeds of many beautiful flowers. But when it bloomed, his garden was filled not just with his chosen flowers but it was also overrun by dandelions. He sought out advice from gardeners all over and tried every method known to get rid of them, but to no avail. Finally, he walked all the way to the capital to speak to the royal gardener at the sheik's palace. The wise old man had counseled many gardeners before and suggested a variety of remedies to expel the dandelions, but Mulla had tried them all. They sat together in silence for some time and finally the gardener looked at Nasrudin and said, "Well, then I suggest you learn to love them."
>
> — Andrew M. Greeley and Mary G. Durkin,
> *The Book of Love: A Treasury Inspired By The Greatest of Virtues*

Have patience with everything unresolved in your heart and try to love the questions themselves as if they were locked rooms or books written in a very foreign language. Don't search for answers now, because you would not be able to live them. And the point is to live everything. Live the questions now. Perhaps then, someday far in the future, you will gradually, without even noticing it, live your way into the answer.

— Rainer Maria Rilke, *Letters to a Young Poet*

Terry Gross: Can you share some of your favorite comments from readers that you've gotten over the years?

Maurice Sendak: Oh, there's so many. Can I give you just one that I really like? It was from a little boy. He sent me a charming card with a little drawing. I loved it. I answer all my children's letters— sometimes very hastily—but this one I lingered over. I sent him a postcard and I drew a picture of a Wild Thing on it. I wrote, "Dear Jim, I loved your card." Then I got a letter back from his mother and she said, "Jim loved your card so much he ate it." That to me was one of the highest compliments I've ever received. He didn't care that it was an original drawing or anything. He saw it, he loved it, he ate it.

— Sy Safransky,
Sunbeams: Sages, Saints and Lovers Celebrate the Human Heart

A Spinning Top—
One Whole Mindful Experience

Daniel Rouse

Having recently returned from a five-day mindfulness retreat at the Blue Cliff Monastery with Thich Nhat Hanh and about 500 others, I walked into my second-grade classroom with great hopes and dreams. I had my bell in hand, my new Zen story books, and a commitment to help the children slow down and focus. I decided to tell the kids about my time away and that I would explain my absence by saying that I had been at a gathering where I was learning about paying attention. Simple enough.

During our morning time on the rug altogether, I talked about being at a Buddhist monastery and about the retreat, and I spoke about mindfulness and being present and attentive. The children all agreed that it was a good idea to pay attention when you are trying to learn about something. They decided that it would be hard to learn something if you didn't really look at it and think about it. The group also concluded that it makes sense to be alert to one's world if one truly wants to experience something through sight, sound, touch, smell, or taste. It would be hard to eat a piece of pizza if you didn't know it was there!

The discussion then turned to how to really see what is in front of you. In my enthusiasm, I came up with an on-the-spot analogy about seeing. I like to paint pictures with words. I tell a lot of stories with lessons. Sometimes I get it right. Sometimes I'm a bit off target. So, I asked the kids to imagine being a spinning top. We talked about what that might be like—particularly if you were trying to look at one thing in one place. You would have to look, spin, look again—look, spin, look—and so on. We all agreed that it would be a challenge to really see something if you only got a series of quick glances interrupted by spinning away over and over. Then I said, "Imagine being a dragonfly who lands on a lily pad in a pond." I asked the children if they thought a dragonfly would "see" the pond better than a spinning top. After a divergent conversation about compound eyes and how they refract light, they began to make sense of my analogy. I was feeling pretty proud of myself as a master teacher when a child pointed out that, in fact, a top spinning on a lily pad in the center of a pond would see the entire pond—all at the same time! How true, we agreed—with each revolution the entire pond would be surveyed and could be taken in as one whole experience.

Through this experience, I learned a number of lessons. First, my second-graders helped me to see that in my efforts to introduce mindfulness, I had not been very mindful myself. My analogy was not really built on solid ground. Comparing my spinning top analogy with the dragonfly imagery was comparing apples to oranges. I had not discerned what it was that the spinning top and the dragonfly were trying to see. Second, and more important, while "seeing" is all well and good, the object of sight is not a given. Generalizations about "seeing" and "experiencing" are not very useful. Assumptions made, but not articulated, can cause confusion. In future lessons designed to help children learn to be more mindful, I had better be certain that I am specific in my goals and that my pedagogy conveys purpose in clear terms. The third lesson was humility. I recognized from the children's observations that mindfulness is not something to be deposited by teachers into the minds of students.

About the Authors

Denise Aldridge, M.S., has taught for 14 years and loves working with students at Friends School in Atlanta. An avid athlete, Denise enjoys judo, yoga, dancing, swimming, hiking, snowboarding and camping. She loves to encourage students' delight and excitement when investigating science, the arts, math, and creative writing. Her mantras are "Treat each other with respect" and "You are what you do every day."

Judy Belasco, B.F.A., a marinescape painter residing in Maine and Philadelphia, taught art in the lower school at Germantown Friends School for 32 years where she co-founded the lower school Quakerism committee and served as its clerk for 10 years. She is an active yoga student and has served as coordinator of regular public yoga programs. She was a founding parent of Project Learn School in Philadelphia.

Hope Blosser, M.Ed., middle school English Teacher at Brooklyn Friends School, has taught for over a decade in various schools, including in central Ethiopia with the Peace Corps, and in public and private schools within the United States. She has been an active practitioner in the Zen community for many years and took lay precepts in 1997. Currently, Hope practices and teaches adults about Zen meditation at the Boundless Mind Zendo in Brooklyn, New York.

Barry Blumenfeld, M.A., is the dance educator at Friends Seminary School in Manhattan, where he has built the dance program over the past 10 years. He is an adjunct professor at New York University and serves on the board of the New York State Dance Education Association. Barry is also a certified yoga instructor and the artistic director of the dance company, TapFusion.

Richard Brady, M.S., is a writer and an educational consultant with Minding Your Life, an organization that helps educators and schools wishing to incorporate mindfulness practices to enhance learning and promote more centered, less stressful life. His publications include: "Schooled in the Moment: Introducing Mindfulness to Students and Teachers," *Independent School* (2004) and "Learning to Stop, Stopping to Learn: Discovering the Contemplative Dimension in Education," *Journal of Transformative Education* (2007).

Janet Chance, M.Ed., began her teaching career at Friends School Tokyo, where she used drama and music to teach English to Japanese students. She now serves as the Lower School Director at William Penn Charter School. Janet has long held a keen interest in studying how communities support spiritual and ethical growth. She is currently exploring possibilities for creating a "spiraling clearness curriculum" for Lower School students.

Christie Duncan-Tessmer, Associate Secretary for Program and Religious Life for Philadelphia Yearly Meeting of the Religious Society of Friends, has a common thread through her work — the task of creating space for multigenerational communities to explore and experience what it means to live together from the center of God. She has served children and their communities in a variety of Quaker organizations and schools and has worked with child witnesses and victims of violence in social service settings.

Sumi Loundon Kim, M.A., M.T.S., has edited two anthologies, *Blue Jean Buddha: Voices of Young Buddhists* (Wisdom, 2001) and *The Buddha's Apprentices: More Voices of Young Buddhists* (Wisdom, 2005). She was Associate Director at the Barre Center for Buddhist Studies in Barre, MA. Sumi teaches mindfulness practice to young people both in Asia and America, and has written extensively on the young adult encounter of Buddhism and meditation.

Rebecca Martin-Scull, M.A., C.P.C.R.T., teaches mindfulness, Quaker studies, comparative religion and library skills to students from preschool through middle school at Media-Providence Friends School. She has taught and supervised public school special education programs and maintains a cognitive rehabilitation practice specializing in mindfulness, brain-awareness work, and organizational skills. Becky teaches piano using a highly cognitive method. An officer for the Society of Cognitive Rehabilitation, she reviews therapists seeking Certification in Cognitive Rehabilitation Therapy.

Eric Mayer, M.Div., is Chair of Religious Studies and a member of the art department at Westtown School. He teaches several courses there, including world religions and "The Contemplative Experience." The photos on the cover and throughout *Tuning In* are from student mandala projects, composed in Eric's world religions class, a required junior-year course.

Irene McHenry, Ph.D., Executive Director of the Friends Council on Education, was founding Head of Delaware Valley Friends School and co-founded Greenwood Friends School and Fielding Graduate University's EdD program. She serves on the boards of Council for American Private Education, Haverford College, and Friends Education Fund. She co-authored *Readings on Quaker Pedagogy* (2004) and *Governance Handbook for Friends Schools* (2002). Irene has taught mindfulness to children and adults in independent schools across the country.

Kimberly Post Rowe, M.Ed., is founder and Executive Director of Five Seeds, a not-for-profit organization dedicated to reducing the impact of stress on individuals and communities through education and awareness. She teaches in private and community colleges in Maine, teaches mindfulness to teens and people living with cancer, and freelances as a copy editor. Her first book, *A Settled Mind*, was published in 2007. Her upcoming books include *Contemplative Ecology* and a foray into junior fiction.

Chip Poston, M.A., served as Religion Department Head at George School for 20 years. From 1993-1996 he was a peace development worker for the Mennonite Central Committee in Jerusalem, where he has returned with student and adult groups five times in the last decade. Chip worked with the Young Friends at George School in developing the Meeting for Worship Orientation Program from 1996-2007. He is also the author of *Minding the Light: Forty-five Lessons for Teaching About Quakerism* (available via www.friendscouncil.org).

Daniel Rouse, M.A., teaches second grade at Germantown Friends School. He has taught for more than 25 years and delights in his work to nurture imagination, empathy, and compassion.

Mary Scattergood, M.S., teaches second grade at Friends School Haverford. Mary has taught at Abington Friends and public school in Vermont. She collaborated with teachers and professors at Dartmouth College to develop the course, "Mentoring New Teachers." She is a meditation leader at the Philadelphia Meditation Center. She is also part of a ministries group at Main Line Unitarian Church. She teaches mindfulness practices to her second graders at Friends School Haverford.

Marcy Seitel, M.A., recently became Middle School Head at Oakwood Friends School and is working with teachers to develop mindfulness practices for their students. Previously, she was Middle School Principal at Thornton Friends School and a teacher at Friends Community School. Marcy adds her interest in mindfulness practices to her years of experience exploring the teaching of conflict resolution, peacemaking, and community building in the schools, especially Friends schools.

Mary B. Minor Sidwell, Director of Development at Olney Friends School, has served in a number of roles at the school over the years. Early in their marriage, Mary and her husband Richard (now Head of School) taught at Olney. They also spent two years at Arthur Morgan School in Celo, North Carolina.

Douglas Tsoi, J.D., has managed a diverse career in law, education and community development. Douglas taught global ethics and sustainability at George School, a Quaker school in Pennsylvania and prior to that, wrote and negotiated contracts as an intellectual property lawyer. Douglas led a cross-sector, collaborative project between Open Meadow Alternative School students and the Portland Schools Foundation to produce a youth video about Portland high school graduation rates.

References

Byrd, Baylor and Parnall, Peter (1974). *Everybody Needs a Rock*. Atheneum.

Byrd, Baylor and Parnall, Peter (1997). *The Other Way to Listen*. Aladdin Paperbacks.

Fothergill, John, in Paul Lacey (1998). *Growing Into Goodness*. Pendle Hill Publications.

Cisneros, Sandra (1991). *The House on Mango Street*. Vintage Contemporaries.

Friends Council on Education (2008). *Advices and Queries for Friends School Community Life*.

Greeley, Andrew and Mary G. Durkin (2004). *The Book of Love: a Treasury Inspired by the Greatest of Virtues*. Forge Books.

Hadley, Abby A. (1972). *We're Going to Meeting for Worship*. Friends General Conference.

Hart, Tobin (2004). "Opening the Contemplative Mind in the Classroom. *Journal of Transformative Education* Vol. 2 No. 1, Sage Publications.

Hays, Kim (1994), *Practicing Virtues: Moral Traditions at Quaker and Military Boarding Schools*. University of California Press.

Hoffman, Jan (1996), *"Clearness Committees and Their Use in Personal Discernment" in Resources for Fostering Vital Friends Meetings*. twelfth month press.

Janoe, Barbara (1988). *Daniel Goes to Meeting*. Family and Life Enrichment.

Kabat-Zinn Jon (2005). *Full Catastrophe Living*. Random House, Inc.

Kabat-Zinn (1994). *Wherever You Go, There You Are*. Hyperion.

Morris, William Barrett (1972). *The Oyster's Secret*. Hubbard Press.

Nhat Hanh, Thich (1996). *The Miracle of Mindfulness*. Beacon Press.

Nhat Hanh, Thich (1988). *The Sun My Heart*. Parallax Press.

Noddings, Nel (2005). *The Challenge to Care in Schools: An Alternative Approach to Education*. Teachers College Press.

Norris, Kathleen (1997). *The Cloister Walk*. Riverhead Books.

Palmer, Parker (1998). *The Courage to Teach: Exploring the Inner Landscape of a Teacher's Life*. Jossey-Bass, Inc.

Palmer, Parker (2000). *Meeting for Learning: Education in a Quaker Context*. Friends Council on Education.

Palmer, Parker, "The Clearness Committee," Center for Courage and Renewal's Web site: www.couragerenewal.org/parker/writings; also see couragerenewal.org

Rilke, Rainer Maria (2004). *Letters to a Young Poet*. W. W. Norton & Company.

Safransky, Sy (1993). *Sunbeams: Sages, Saints and Lovers Celebrate the Human Heart*. North Atlantic Books.

Siegel, Daniel (2007). *The Mindful Brain*. W.W. Norton & Company.

Starmer, Nancy, in Friends Council on Education (2004). *Readings on Quaker Pedagogy*.

Weiss, Andrew (2004). *Beginning Mindfulness: Learning the Way of Awareness*, New World Library.